AlCohOL, dRuG& tObACco UsE

STATISTICS ON

AlCohOL, dRuG& tobACco UsE

A Selection of Statistical Charts, Graphs and Tables About Alcohol, Drug and Tobacco Use From a Variety of Published Sources with Explanatory Comments

Timothy L. Gall and
Daniel M. Lucas, *Editors*

Carl G. Leukefeld, Director
Multidisciplinary Research Center on
Drug and Alcohol Abuse
University of Kentucky,
Contributing Editor

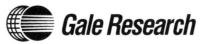

Gale Research

An ITP Infromation/Reference Group Company

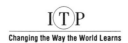

Changing the Way the World Learns

NEW YORK • LONDON • BONN • BOSTON • DETROIT
MADRID • MELBOURNE • MEXICO CITY • PARIS
SINGAPORE • TOKYO • TORONTO • WASHINGTON
ALBANY NY • BELMONT CA • CINCINNATI OH

Eastword Publications Development Inc. Staff
Timothy L. Gall and Daniel M. Lucas, *Editors*

Gale Research Inc. Staff
Donna Wood, *Coordinating Editor*

Mary Beth Trimper, *Production Manager*
Cynthia D. Baldwin, *Product Design Manager*
Barbara J. Yarrow, *Graphic Services Supervisor*
Michelle DiMercurio, *Art Director*

♾™ The paper used in this publication meets the minimum requirements of American National Standard for Information Sciences-Permanence Paper for Printed Library Materials, ANSI Z39.48-1984.

♻ This book is printed on recycled paper that meets Environmental Protection Agency standards.

Copyright © 1996
Gale Research Inc.
835 Penobscot Bldg.
Detroit, MI 48226-4094

Printed in the United States of America

Library of Congress Cataloging-in-Publication Data

Statistics on alcohol, drug and tobacco use : a selection of
statistical charts, graphs, and tables about alcohol, drug, and
tobacco use from a variey of published sources with explanatory
comments / Timothy L. Gall and Daniel L. Lucas, editors.
    p. cm.
  Includes bibliographical references and index.
  ISBN 0-7876-0526-3 (alk. paper)
  1. Drinking of alcoholic beverages--United States--Statistics.
2. Drug abuse--United States--Statistics. 3. Tobacco habit--United
States--Statiistics. I. Gall, Timothy L. II. Lucas, Daniel M.
  HV5292.S73 1995
  362.29' 12' 0973--dc20   95-32413
                                        CIP

 Gale Research Inc., an International Thomson Publishing Company.
ITP logo is a trademark under license.

10 9 8 7 6 5 4 3 2 1

How to use this book

This book presents statistics on alcohol, illegal drug, and tobacco use in the United States. Each of the statistical presentations appears on a two-page spread. The table or graphic containing the statistics is presented on a left-hand page and the explanatory text, the source citation, and contact information appears on the facing right-hand page. Also included in this volume is a general introduction to the problems of alcohol, drug, and tobacco use and a glossary of related terminology. Finally, a thorough index facilitates ease of use.

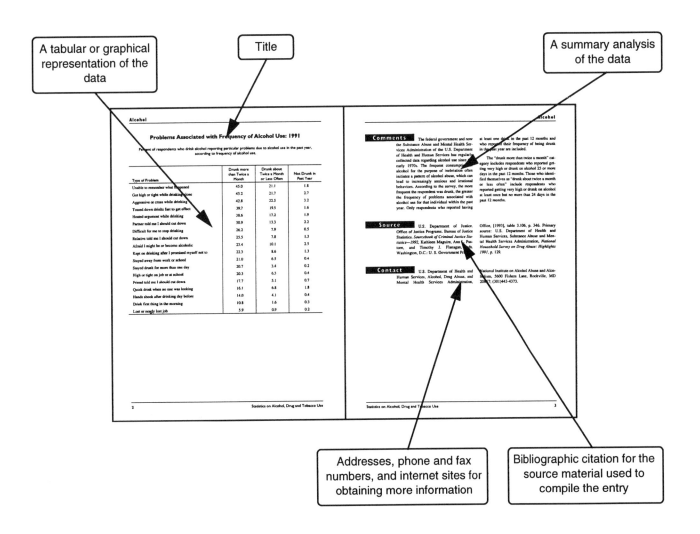

A tabular or graphical representation of the data

Title

A summary analysis of the data

Addresses, phone and fax numbers, and internet sites for obtaining more information

Bibliographic citation for the source material used to compile the entry

Advisory Board

Judith H. Higgins
Director of LRC, Valhalla High School Library, Valhalla, New York

Connie Lawson
Librarian, Maple Heights Regional Library, Cuyahoga County Public Library, Maple Heights, Ohio

Deborah Lee
Librarian, Los Angeles County Public Library, Rowland Heights, California

John Ranahan
Teacher, Lake Ridge Academy, Oberlin, Ohio

Linda Taft
Librarian, Morgantown High School, Morgantown, West Virginia

Lynda C. Tirhi
Librarian, Nimitz High School Library, Irving, Texas

Table of Contents

Introduction ix

ALCOHOL

Problems Associated with Frequency of Alcohol Use: 1991 2
Problems Associated with Alcohol Use by Age Group of Drinker: 1991 4
Consumption of Alcohol by Age Group: 1974–91 6
Demographic Characteristics of Alcohol Users: 1991 8
Past Month Alcohol Use:1974–91 10
Alcohol Use by High School Seniors: 1982–93 12
Drinking and Other Unhealthy Behaviors in Adolescents: 1992 14
Adolescent Drinking and Smoking: 1992 16
Fatal Traffic Injuries Involving Alcohol: 1983–93 18
Motor Vehicle Crash Fatalities by State: 1993 20
Blood Alcohol Concentrations (BACs) of Fatally Injured Drivers: 1993 22
Fatalities in Alcohol-Related Traffic Accidents: 1982–91 24
Alcohol Involvement in Automobile Crashes: 1988–91 26
Lives Saved by Drinking Age Laws and Alcohol-Related
   Youth Fatalities, 1985–93 28
Fatally Injured Drunk Drivers: 1980–93 30
Youth Crash Fatalities and Alcohol: 1982–93 32
Youth Crash Fatality Rate and Alcohol: 1982–93 34
DUI Arrests by Selected Characteristics: 1993 36
Total Arrests for DUI: 1993 38
Arrests for Alcohol-Related Offenses and DUI: 1972–93 40
Arrests for Drunkenness: 1993 42
Drunkenness Arrests in the U.S.: 1993 44
Fatal Workplace Injuries Involving Alcohol: 1992 46
Fetal Alcohol Syndrome Rates: 1979–93 48
Alcohol-Induced Deaths: 1979–92 50

DRUGS

Major Federal Drug Control Legislation:1868–1990 54
World Production of Three Illegal Drug Crops: 1987–91 56
Worldwide Production of Cocaine: 1992 and 1993 58
Worldwide Production of Opium: 1988–93 60
Worldwide Production of Marijuana: 1988–93 62
Worldwide Production of Hashish: 1988–93 64
Drugs Smuggled into the U.S.: 1986 66
Individuals Reporting Illegal Drug Use: 1993 68
Cocaine Use and Overall Illegal Drug Use: 1979–93 70
Estimated Cocaine and Heroin Users: 1988–93 72
Annual Cocaine Consumption: 1972–92 74
Drug Use Among High School Seniors: 1991–94 76
Effects of Illegal Drugs 78
Drug Ranking Schedule of the DEA 80

Contents

Drug Use by Arrested Persons: 1991 82

Sampling of Past Month Drug Use: 1992 84

Liquor and Marijuana Use Among Youth and their Role
  in Violent Behavior: 1993–94 86

Young Adults' Past Month Drug Use: 1974–91 88

Steroid Use by High School Seniors: 1989–94 90

Drug Use by U.S. Military Personnel: 1992 92

Drug Testing Programs in Private Business: 1989 94

Deaths in the Workplace Involving Drugs: 1992 96

Drug-Related Murders in the U.S.: 1986–93 98

THC Content of Seized Marijuana: 1975–90 100

Drug-Related Arrests: 1988–93 102

Drug Use During Crimes: 1990 104

Regional Distribution of Drug Law Violation Arrests: 1981–1993 106

How Drug Cases Are Handled: 1992 108

Offenses for which Prisoners are Admitted to State Prisons: 1982–92 110

Inmates in State Prisons and Proportion of Drug Offenders: 1979–92 112

Demographic Characteristics of Convicted Drug Felons: 1992 114

Average Lengths of Drug Felony Sentences: 1992 116

Felony Convictions in State Courts: 1992 118

Federal Drug Convictions: 1985–92 120

Federal Drug Control Spending: 1982–93 122

Federal Drug Control Spending by Function: 1995–96 124

State and Local Drug Control Spending: 1991 126

Drug Enforcement by Local and State Law Enforcement Agencies: 1990 128

Multiagency Drug Enforcement Task Force Participants: 1990 130

Federal Seizures of Marijuana, Cocaine, and Heroin: 1989–93 132

Land and Marine Seizures of Marijuana and Cocaine: 1976–92 134

Seizures of Illegal Drug Laboratories: 1975–91 136

International Drug Seizures: 1989–93 138

Destruction of Cannabis Plants in the States: 1982–90 140

Cannabis Eradication Efforts: 1990 142

State and Local Narcotics Enforcement: 1990 144

Asset Seizure by the DEA: 1992 146

Federal Asset Forfeiture Funds: 1986–90 148

Monthly Drug-Related Personal Income Amounts 150

Total U.S. Expenditures on Illicit Drugs: 1988–93 152

Retail Prices per Gram of Cocaine: 1988–93 154

Retail Prices per Gram of Heroin: 1988–93 156

Retail Price per Gram of Cocaine by Region: 1986-91 158

Wholesale Prices for Marijuana: 1991 160

Wholesale Cocaine Prices: 1991 162

Costs to Society from Illegal Drug Use 164

Emergency Room Episodes and Drug Use: 1988–93 166

Drug-Induced Deaths by Gender: 1979–92 168

Reasons for Emergency Room Visits: 1993 170

Census of Clients in Alcohol and/or Drug Abuse Treatment: 1980–92 172

Drug Abuse Treatment: 1989–96 174

Drug Treatment Costs: 1989 176

TOBACCO

Per Capita Yearly Consumption of Cigarettes: 1900–94 180
Cigarette Smokers by State, 35 Years Old and Over: 1990 182
Cigarette Smokers by Race, Education, Age, and Income: 1992 184
Women Smokers Aged 18–44: 1987–92 186
Cigarette Smoking by High School Seniors: 1975–94 188
Cigarette Smoking by Youths Aged 12–21: 1992 190
Smokeless Tobacco Use by Teenagers: 1986–94 192
Prevalence of Selected Reasons for Using Cigarettes: 1993 194
Nicotine Withdrawal Symptoms Reported by Teenagers: 1993 196
Costs of Medical Care for Smoking-Related Sickness: 1987 198
Potential Years of Life Lost Due to Smoking: 1990 200
Deaths Attributed to Smoking: 1990 202
Relative Risks Attributable to Smoking: 1990 204
Results of Surveys on Prohibiting or Restricting Smoking: 1993 206
Results of Surveys on Effective Strategies to Prevent Teenage Smoking: 1993 208

Glossary. 211
Index. 221

Introduction

by Carl G. Leukefeld, Director
Multidisciplinary Research Center on Drug and Alcohol Abuse,
University of Kentucky

Statistics on Alcohol, Drug and Tobacco Use is an accurate and easy-to-use reference text for students and others who are interested in information on alcohol, tobacco, and other drugs. This reference book provides data with table and graphic presentations which are combined with descriptions to explain trends related to substance use, abuse, and dependency in the United States. References are also given at the end of each section that can be consulted if additional information is needed. These data are a beginning for the serious student, for there is an expanding body of literature about alcohol, tobacco, and drugs available.

Alcohol and other drugs have been used as mood-altering substances throughout history; they filter our senses and help us feel better. These substances have also been used to block unpleasant people, situations, and events from our consciousness. For many Americans, however, substance abuse becomes an addiction that not only affects the well being of the individual user, but also the well being of society at large. Consequently, Americans have always had, and continue to have, an interest in addiction. However, America's response to addiction has changed over time. Attitudes and opinions are constantly influenced by politics, celebrity involvement, and crime. In addition, we are influenced by the way substance abuse issues are presented in the media (TV, radio, and newspapers). These forces affect our attitudes, and ultimately our approach to dealing with the problem.

One thing to keep in mind when studying alcohol and other drug use is that different people can look at substance abuse in very different ways. For example, substance abuse treatment providers are most concerned with helping alcohol and drug abusers stop abusing substances. Their goal is to stop patients enrolled in drug treatment programs from using drugs. Police and law enforcement officials, however, look at the drug problem differently. They focus on crimes related to drug use, and stopping the sales of illegal drugs. Their efforts include minimum/maximum sentencing laws for drug abusers. The result of these policies is American jails and prisons overflowing with drug users who commit crimes. From another point of view, school officials focus on the drug problem as an educational issue. Teachers are interested in developing and delivering drug education programs. However, when school officials are asked about drug use, they are usually quick to deny the possibility that there is a drug problem in their schools.

Ultimately, it is up to the policy makers in our local, state, and federal governments to reconcile these diverse approaches, and to allocate scarce resources to solving the problem. Too often, however, policy makers focus on "quick fixes" for the substance abuse problem. The remedies taken frequently parallel public opinion polls. For example, as the public's attitudes towards drug use have hardened, policy makers have been quick to change their emphasis from treatment for drug abusers, to law enforcement strategies to reduce drug availability. At the same time, public health officials have become more involved and more vocal in the drug abuse debate. They advocate distributing needles and condoms—together with advice on the importance of abstinence—to people who inject drugs. Their purpose is to reduce the spread of HIV among injectors. This is because injectors make up about one-third of all persons with AIDS, and are a major source leading to the heterosexual spread of HIV, a serious and expensive public health problem. The public's perception of which approach is most effective is always an important factor in shaping public policy.

This ongoing debate on how best to deal with America's substance abuse problems continues to influence public perception and, therefore, public policy. Recent policy changes have included recommendations to legalize drugs. Tobacco, on the other hand, is now being considered an addictive substance for possible regulation by the federal Food and Drug Administration. However, tobacco—although an addictive and deadly substance for users—is a cash crop for southern farmers, and therefore a political "hot potato" for southern congressmen. With so many different approaches being advocated, a well-informed public is critical to finding the most effective and appropriate solutions to the complex and challenging problem of substance abuse.

The Nature of Abuse

The drug section of this book focuses on unlawful drug use and drug abuse rather than on lawful drug use. Lawful or prescription drugs are prescribed by physicians for medical purposes. When many of us think about drugs, we tend to focus on drugs of abuse. However, there are a number of people who could not function or live without prescribed medications. These medications include drugs for hypertension, insulin for diabetics, thyroid for those who do not produce enough thyroid, and many more.

We also need to keep in mind that some substances, particularly alcohol and tobacco, have been used in traditional celebrations, and are part of many of our lives. For example, most of us have heard the phrases "I'll drink to that!" or "Let's toast to our success!" after a milestone has been reached. However, some are unable to partake of traditionally used substances in moderation. For them, use progresses to abuse, and abuse leads to dependency or addiction. Once an individual becomes dependent or addicted, that person has a chronic and relapsing disorder, even if he or she has voluntarily chosen to quit taking substances. That is to say that the person must always be mindful of his or her dependency, and realize that addiction will not just go away. This person is always at risk to return to abusing substances. It has been said that it is easy to stop, but it is most difficult to stop and not use again. A person who has stopped but started again usually goes back to using the drug at the same level as before, often with tragic results.

Statistical Reliability

Drug, alcohol, and tobacco data are usually collected and reported using three measures which are consistently found in the literature on these subjects. (1) *Current use,* which is the use of a substance in the past

thirty days. (2) *Past year use,* which is the use of a substance in the past year. (3) *Lifetime use,* which is any use of a substance in a person's life. Lifetime use for each substance is usually the highest level reported, followed by past year use, and then current use. This is because a user will always have used more drugs in a lifetime than during the past year or 30 days.

An important point to keep in mind when using the data in this volume is that most of the information presented is based on survey data which was collected using face-to-face interviews and telephone interviews. Consequently, most of the data on the use and abuse of substances are self-reported and not confirmed by laboratory tests.

There have been questions raised about collecting self-reported information concerning illegal activities, and drug use specifically. Many researches have questioned the reliability of self-reported data by insisting that respondents may be reluctant to admit engaging in an illegal activity, and therefore may not answer the questions honestly or completely. Other researchers, however, point out that this information is collected in a confidential manner and individuals' names are not used. In addition, much of the information is collected anonymously; names are never asked, used, or collected. With the protection of confidentiality, it is assumed that people will talk honestly and openly about their use of substances. They know the information they provide is confidential, frequently anonymous, and used only for research purposes.

In addition to interviews, there are many situations where bodily fluids are collected to determine current use of a specific substance. This is often the case where a person has been taken into custody by the police, is applying for a job, or working in an industry where other peoples lives may be at risk, as in the case of a school bus driver. Bodily fluids that can be checked for drugs include urine samples, which are collected and analyzed for substances by a laboratory using thin layer chromatography or glass chromatography. On-site testing kits are also used to analyze urine for drugs. The advantage of on-site testing is that there is an immediate response for the presence or absence of a drug or drugs. Breath is used to test for the presence of alcohol as are blood samples. Hair can be collected and analyzed to determine the presence of a drug, and when the drug was used. Although an effective technique, collecting bodily fluids is controversial. Some people have questioned the appropriateness of using these techniques for research, as part of screening for job entry for certain professions, and to maintain a person's job. In addition, many Americans resent the invasion of privacy that accompanies mandatory drug testing. Consequently, these practices continue to be debated by policy makers and members of the public alike.

Some of the data in this volume are given with confidence intervals, or the margin of error of the survey, to describe the entire population from which the sample was selected. The margin of error can be dependent upon a number of factors, including the fact that the survey sample selected was limited in size. A confidence interval usually describes the range that would account for 95% of the population being described and is expressed as a plus and minus of a specific percentage which is statistically determined. For a 95% confidence interval, the actual rate could vary by 10% with the confidence interval expressed at 5% more and 5% less than the actual percentage reported from the survey.

Illegal Drugs

America's efforts to control drugs have shifted between supply reduction initiatives and demand reduction initiatives. Supply initiatives involve stopping the supply of drugs to the end user. Demand initiatives involve efforts aimed at decreasing the end user's demand for drugs.

Supply reduction has generally focused on drug enforcement strategies to stop drug distribution networks like those made famous in the movie *The French Connection.* Supply reduction also includes crop replacement programs. In many poor countries, illegal drugs are an important cash crop and an integral part of the local economy. Crop replacement programs encourage farmers to grow legal crops instead of illegal ones. Although strategies designed to disrupt the economic structure of drug distribution have been effective, enforcement activities by agencies like the Drug Enforcement Administration (DEA) are more commonly used to reduce the supply of drugs. These activities rely on arrests, seizures, and punishment to discourage drug supply and distribution.

Demand reduction activities on the other hand, focus on providing education, intervention, and treatment services to prevent or stop substance abuse. These policies are designed to stop the demand for drugs.

Recently there has been considerable discussion among policy makers on whether America should pursue policies that stop the supply of drugs or policies that reduce the demand for drugs. As American voters have elected more conservative policy makers, the United States has shifted emphasis from demand reduction techniques to supply reduction techniques aimed at stopping drugs at the source of supply. Although it may seem obvious that a balanced approach to drug supply and demand reduction is needed, political events continue to redirect resources away from education and treatment. Americans want a quick solution to the problem of substance abuse, but the chronic and relapsing nature of substance abuse as a disorder makes quick solutions ineffective.

Although there has been a recent shift from education and treatment solutions to enforcement solutions, many policy makers recognize the need for a balanced approach. Clearly, a person can not be addicted to an illegal substance without the substance. Controls are needed to limit supply and availability. These controls and limitations include laws related to the sale and distribution of prescribed drugs through a physician, age limitations related to the sale of tobacco and alcohol, and regulation of the hours for selling alcohol and of the age for obtaining a drivers license. But treatment and prevention/education interventions are also necessary.

Regardless of which strategies are being pursued, all advocates rely on drug use statistics to formulate their positions. Data frequently cited when analyzing America's drug problem include Drug Use Forecasting (DUF) data collected in U.S. jails and lock ups, data from the National Household Survey, and data collected in the Senior High School Survey. Some key findings from these and other surveys are presented below. Taken together, the data paints a vivid picture of America's drug use problem.

- The total U.S. expenditure on illicit drugs decreased by 24% from 1988 to 1993—from $65.7 billion in 1988 to $50.1 billion in 1993, a $16.5 billion reduction. The level of expenditures for cocaine decreased from about $42 billion to about $32 billion. For heroin, the level of expenditures decreased from almost $12 billion to $7.4 billion. Expenditures for marijuana remained the same at about $9 billion. Expenditures for other drugs decreased from about $3 billion to about $2 billion.

- Drug use data confirmed by urine tests for eleven drugs collected in 24 city jails and lock ups show that in 1991, men tested positive for any drug at a level which ranged from 36% to 75%. The percent of women testing positive for any drug ranged from 45% to 79% in these 24 U.S. cities. Stated differently, about 4 to 7 of every 10 men who were booked and almost 5 to 8 of every 10 women who were booked in 1991 tested positive for an illegal drug.

- Data from the 1993 National Household Survey revealed that over one-third (37%)—or more than 77 million people—in U.S. households 12 years of age and older reported use of an illicit drug during their lifetime. Seventy million people reported use of marijuana, while 23 million had tried cocaine, 18 million had used hallucinogens, 4 million had tried crack-cocaine, and more than 2 million had tried heroin. Current use—defined as use within the past 30 days—of any illicit drug was at 5.6%. Overall, however, reported drug use was found to be decreasing among household residents. In addition, an overall decrease in both casual and heavy heroin use as well as cocaine use was noted from 1988 to 1993. The only exception was an increase in heavy heroin use from 1992 to 1993.

- The Senior High School Survey data are useful in helping to understand the level of drug use among students. The Senior High School Survey asks a representative sample of seniors about their drug use. When these data from 1991 to 1994 are examined, it shows that drug use among seniors increased steadily. However, drug use among seniors has been steadily decreasing from the high of 54% in 1979 to a low of 40% in 1992.

- Hospital emergency room episodes increased about 14% from over 403,000 in 1988 to 466,897 in 1993. These emergency episodes are defined as episodes representing a single occurrence where the use of a drug was revealed or detected. In 1993,

the drug-related reasons given for going to emergency rooms were: overdose, 53%; chronic effects, 11%; unexpected reactions,12%; seeking detoxification, 10%; withdrawal, 2%; and other/unknown reasons, 12%. Deaths by drug-induced causes increased from 1979 to 1992. For females the increase was 14% (from 3,445 to 3,937) and for males it more than doubled (from 3,656 to 7,766).

- Private businesses are concerned about drug abuse. In 1989, about 3% of businesses reported that they had established drug testing programs. Less than one percent of retail trade business had established testing programs, compared to almost 22% of companies engaged in communications and public utilities businesses.

- There is a substantial amount of data available on drug production, availability, and drug seizures. For example, world production of opium, which is used to make heroin, increased from 1987 to 1990. Coca leaf production, which is used to make cocaine, also increased, with several South American countries—Bolivia, Columbia, Peru—being the major producers. Burma, Afghanistan, Laos, Pakistan, Mexico, Thailand, Columbia, Lebanon, and Guatemala are estimated to be the major producers of opium. Mexico has the greatest potential for international marijuana production, followed by Columbia and Belize. Lebanon, Pakistan, Afghanistan, and Morocco have the greatest potential for hashish production.

- The statistic for drug-related arrests as a percent of total U.S. arrests has fluctuated from 8.4% in 1983 to 8% in 1993, with a high in that period of 9.5% in 1989. However, the percent of arrests for U.S. drug law violations increased from 22% in 1981 to 30% in 1993. While all drug offenses are investigated, of the number persons prosecuted in 1993, 65% were convicted, and of those convicted, 53% were sent to prison and 10% were placed on probation.

- While the number of state prisoners increased by almost three times from 1979 to 1992, the number of inmates incarcerated for drug offenses increased by an even larger amount, from 6% to 22%. Sentencing for drug possession was shorter than for trafficking. At the federal level, from 1985 to 1992, drug convictions for drug distribution increased by

103%. For that same time period the number of drug manufacturing cases prosecuted increased by 349%. Overall, there was an 82% increase in the number of all types of drug offenses.

- Depending on the bulk and weight of an illegal drug, smugglers generally use three approaches to bring drugs into the U.S.: aircraft is used for most heroin brought into the U.S., while vessels and some vehicles are used for most marijuana and cocaine. During the years 1989 to 1993, it is estimated that 87% of all international drug seizures were for marijuana/hashish, 12% were for cocaine, and 1% for poppy/opium. Asset seizures by the Drug Enforcement Administration for 1992 totaled almost $878 million.

- Along with an increase in arrests related to drugs and drug seizures, the number of persons in treatment for alcohol and drug abuse, based on a one-day census, went from 473,556 in 1980 to 944,990 in 1992. This is almost double. This increase was largest in the 21 to 44 age group at 59%.

Alcohol

In the U.S., alcohol is a legal drug for persons 21 years of age and over. Although legal, alcohol can cause behavioral and health problems when persons drink to excess. Some of the more serious problems associated with alcohol abuse include accidents at home, at work, and while driving an automobile. Many of these accidents affect not only the drinker, but those around the person as well. Much data has been collected to show trends and changes in accident levels. These data help policy makers focus resources on programs directed at reducing the number of accidents and other problems related to the consumption of alcohol. Some of the more important insights into the problem of alcohol abuse in America include the following:

- About 40% of drinkers who report being drunk more than twice per month experience serious problems associated with their drinking. Of the 40% who are drunk twice a month, 45% reported being unable to remember what happened while they were drunk, 43% got high or tight while drinking alone, and 43% became aggressive or cross while drinking. Heavy drinkers in the 18 to 25 age

group generally reported the highest percent of problems. These problems included being unable to remember what happened; being aggressive or cross while drinking; tossing down drinks fast to get the effect; having heated arguments while drinking; and staying drunk for more than one day.

- The consumption of alcohol by those 12 to 17 years old decreased from 54% in 1974 to 46% in 1991. However, consumption of alcohol by those 18 to 25 years old increased from 82% in 1974 to 90% in 1991. In addition, alcohol consumption for those 26 years old and older increased from 73% in 1974 to 89% in 1991.

- Each year about 17,500 deaths from vehicle crashes involve drugs or alcohol. Overall, fatal traffic accidents involving alcohol decreased from 46% in 1983 to 36% in 1993. The greatest decrease was for motorcyclists (13%) while the smallest decrease was for pedestrians (3%). From 1988 to 1991, the percent of automobile crashes involving alcohol remained about the same (6 to 7%). Still, automobile accidents involving alcohol or drugs are the leading cause of death among persons under 25 years of age.

- Changes in drinking age laws that increase the minimum age to 21 have proven to save lives. From 1975 to 1984 data shows that over 5,500 lives were saved. By 1985 that number had increased to over 6,200.

- From 1982 to 1993 alcohol-related crash fatalities for 15 to 20 year old Americans decreased by 44%, from almost 5,400 to about 2,400. However, during that same period, the number of non-alcohol related crash fatalities increased from 3,128 to 3,541.

- For a variety of reasons, including better reporting and better detection, fetal alcohol syndrome (FAS) cases increased from a rate of 1 per 10,000 births in 1974 to 6.7 per 10,000 births in 1993. FAS can be prevented if women do not drink when they are pregnant.

- In 1992, the number of fatal workplace injuries involving alcohol were highest for homicides, followed by highway accidents, transportation accidents, harmful exposures, falls, suicide, and contact with an object.

Tobacco

Tobacco use, whether in the smokeable form (cigarettes, cigars, and pipe tobacco) or smokeless form (chewing tobacco and snuff) is related to premature deaths. That is to say that people who use tobacco, especially cigarettes, will die earlier on the average than those who do not. In fact, the U.S. Public Health Service has advised Americans for a number of years that cigarette smoking is the single most preventable cause of premature deaths in the United States. It is estimated that cigarette smoking is responsible for between 300,000 to 400,000 deaths in the United States each year. Even with the large number of deaths attributed to tobacco, it is estimated that 48 million people over 18 years of age continue to smoke. This represents over one-quarter (26.5%) of the U.S. population over 18 years of age. Although public awareness campaigns warning of the dangers of smoking have caused a decline in smoking over the past decade, an increase in smoking was registered in the 18 to 24 age group in 1992. This increase has been related to increases in targeted advertising by tobacco companies. It is a clear indication that tobacco continues to adversely affect the health of Americans.

Smoking is more common among men than women, and specifically American Indian/Alaskan Natives males. It is also more prevalent among those with less education, and is highest for people living at the poverty level. In 1992 it was estimated that 27% (14.3 million) of all women aged 18–44 were smokers. This decreased from 30% in 1987 to 26% in 1991. Women who smoke, like men, have a greater risk of developing lung cancer and chronic pulmonary disease. Women who smoke are also at risk for complications related to lower birth weight infants and infant mortality during pregnancy.

As with adult smokers, cigarette smoking among high school seniors has declined since 1976, when most drug use peaked among teenagers. The percent of daily users decreased from 29% in 1976 to 19% in 1994. However, from 1992 to 1994 there was a slight increase in cigarette smoking, with a 2% increase in "daily use." Although slight, any increase in cigarette consumption among high school seniors is a worrisome trend worth watching.

Among Americans 12 to 21 years of age, 40% indicated that they did not smoke, while 27% stated they were current smokers, and 29% reported they were experimenters. In addition, smokeless tobacco in the forms of chewing tobacco and snuff, has become more popular among young males. The percent of smokeless tobacco use among males 18–24 increased from 2% in 1970 to 10% in 1991.

Unfortunately, as young smokers eventually learn, having once started, it is difficult to stop smoking. Having trouble quitting is related to the frequency and intensity of the need for nicotine. Nicotine is the addictive substance found in cigarettes and other tobacco products. The more a person smokes, the more that person's body becomes dependent on nicotine, and the harder it is to quit. Over 90% of young adults who smoke tried their first cigarette before they were 20 years of age. When young people first start to smoke, they report finding the experience relaxing. However those who continue to smoke, and smoke more, report smoking as being addictive, since it is difficult for steady smokers to quit smoking.

It needs to be emphasized that American cigarette smokers smoke lots of cigarettes. In 1994 cigarette smokers smoked 480 billion cigarettes. Put another way, cigarette smokers buy about 24 billion packs of cigarettes each year, which is almost the same amount as in 1960. However, the greatest use of cigarettes occurred in 1981 when 640 billion cigarettes were smoked. This grew from 2.5 billion cigarettes smoked in 1900.

Eventually, habitual cigarette use takes its toll on a person's health and on the nation's health care system. Using 1990 data, the death rate per 100,000 population attributed to smoking ranged from of 218 per 100,000 in Utah to the high of 478 per 100,000 in Nevada. Medical costs related to smoking are substantial and represented 7.1% of all 1987 U.S. health care expenditures.

The magnitude of the problems caused by smoking has not been lost on the American public. According to recent survey information, Americans favor restricting tobacco use in public places including bars, restaurants, private work sites, government buildings, and hospitals.

Cities have ordinances which prohibit smoking in public areas, office buildings, and places where people congregate. An eight-state study in 1993 presented the following strategies that were reported to be perceived as being effective by at least half of all respondents: keeping teenagers from smoking by banning smoking on school grounds, banning all cigarette advertising, strongly enforcing laws, banning all cigarette vending machines, and increasing the price of cigarettes.

Summary

What these data indicate is the high level of alcohol, drug, and tobacco use in the United States. Although not the highest recorded use in American history, the use is at levels that are unacceptable for most Americans. This overview of statistical data suggests that Americans use a variety of illegal substances in different ways to alter mood and perception. When two legal drugs—alcohol and tobacco—are examined, it is clear that their addictive qualities take a toll on Americans and are a drain on our health care resources.

Drugs of abuse are plentiful in the U.S. criminal justice system, with high levels of use reported by prisoners as well as those who come into contact with jails and lock ups. A large number of persons are now arrested for drug violations and are currently incarcerated for crimes associated with drug abuse and dependency. Some of these arrestees are criminals who use drugs, while others are drug users who commit crimes to obtain drugs. We need to do a better job of distinguishing between these kinds of motivations.

An overall conclusion, based on the information presented in this volume, is that Americans need to pay consistent attention to substance use, abuse, and dependency. The United States needs to provide a balanced approach to decreasing the amount of drugs coming into our country. We also need to provide prevention and treatment services for those who are substance abusers and dependent upon substances. In addition, we need to be mindful of the fact that we all want quick fixes to the substance abuse problem. However, we need to realize that quick fixes can produce other problems.

AlCohOL

Problems Associated with Frequency of Alcohol Use: 1991

Percent of respondents who drink alcohol reporting particular problems due to alcohol use in the past year, according to frequency of alcohol use.

Type of Problem	Drunk more than Twice a Month	Drunk about Twice a Month or Less Often	Not Drunk in Past Year
Unable to remember what happened	45.0	21.1	1.8
Got high or tight while drinking alone	43.2	21.7	2.7
Aggressive or cross while drinking	42.8	22.5	3.2
Tossed down drinks fast to get effect	39.7	19.5	1.6
Heated argument while drinking	38.6	17.2	1.9
Partner told me I should cut down	30.9	13.3	2.2
Difficult for me to stop drinking	26.2	7.9	0.5
Relative told me I should cut down	25.5	7.8	1.3
Afraid I might be or become alcoholic	23.4	10.1	2.5
Kept on drinking after I promised myself not to	22.3	8.6	1.3
Stayed away from work or school	21.0	6.5	0.4
Stayed drunk for more than one day	20.7	3.4	0.2
High or tight on job or at school	20.3	6.3	0.4
Friend told me I should cut down	17.7	5.1	0.7
Quick drink when no one was looking	16.1	6.8	1.8
Hands shook after drinking day before	14.0	4.1	0.4
Drink first thing in the morning	10.8	1.6	0.3
Lost or nearly lost job	5.9	0.9	0.2

Comments The federal government and now the Substance Abuse and Mental Health Services Administration of the U.S. Department of Health and Human Services has regularly collected data regarding alcohol use since the early 1970s. The frequent consumption of alcohol for the purpose of inebriation often initiates a pattern of alcohol abuse. This can lead to increasingly anxious and irrational behaviors. According to the survey, the more frequent the respondent was drunk, the greater the frequency of problems associated with alcohol use for that individual. Only respondents who reported having at least one drink in the past 12 months and who reported their frequency of being drunk are included.

The "drunk more than twice a month" category includes respondents who reported getting very high or drunk on alcohol 25 or more days in the past 12 months. Those who identified themselves as "drunk about twice a month or less often" include respondents who reported getting very high or drunk on alcohol at least once but no more than 24 days in the past 12 months.

Source U.S. Department of Justice. Office of Justice Programs. Bureau of Justice Statistics. *Sourcebook of Criminal Justice Statistics—1992,* Kathleen Maguire, Ann L. Pastore, and Timothy J. Flanagan, eds. Washington, D.C.: U. S. Government Printing Office, [1993], table 3.106, p. 346. Primary source: U.S. Department of Health and Human Services, Substance Abuse and Mental Health Services Administration, *National Household Survey on Drug Abuse: Highlights 1991*, p. 129.

Contact U.S. Department of Health and Human Services, Alcohol, Drug Abuse, and Mental Health Services Administration, National Institute on Alcohol Abuse and Alcoholism, 5600 Fishers Lane, Rockville, MD 20857; (301)443-4373.

Problems Associated with Alcohol Use by Age Group of Drinker: 1991

Percent of respondents who drink alcohol reporting particular problems due to alcohol use in the past year, according to age group.

Type of Problem	Total all Ages	12–17 Yrs.	18–25 Yrs.	26–34 Yrs.	35 Yrs. and Older
Unable to remember what happened	11.7	14.5	22.2	13.1	7.5
Got high or tight while drinking alone	11.0	11.3	14.2	14.4	8.6
Aggressive or cross while drinking	10.5	22.2	22.5	10.7	5.4
Tossed down drinks fast to get effect	9.5	22.9	23.8	10.1	3.3
Heated argument while drinking	9.0	11.8	19.2	9.5	5.3
Partner told me I should cut down	7.5	9.0	9.6	7.7	6.7
Difficult for me to stop drinking	6.3	13.0	8.0	7.0	4.7
Relative told me I should cut down	5.0	8.8	7.1	5.3	3.8
Afraid I might be or become alcoholic	4.9	6.6	7.7	5.0	3.9
Kept on drinking after I promised myself not to	4.5	9.1	8.5	6.0	2.1
Stayed away from work or school	4.4	22.4	6.0	2.4	2.7
Stayed drunk for more than one day	3.8	5.2	10.6	3.9	1.4
High or tight on job or at school	3.6	10.1	8.8	3.5	1.3
Friend told me I should cut down	3.3	7.2	5.6	2.9	2.3
Quick drink when no one was looking	2.6	5.1	5.9	2.6	1.4
Hands shook after drinking day before	2.5	4.0	5.2	2.1	1.7
Drink first thing in the morning	1.4	1.6	1.	1.5	1.4
Lost or nearly lost job	0.8	0.3	0.8	0.9	0.8

Comments The problems associated with alcohol use vary in frequency according to age. This survey, sponsored by the National Institute on Drug Abuse, randomly surveyed households across the United States to measure the prevalence of alcohol abuse. The problems described here are some of the typical indications that someone may have an alcohol abuse problem.

Alcohol abuse causes personal long-term physical health risks. The behaviors associated with alcohol abuse may also create immediate conditions hazardous to others (e.g., driving under the influence, the role of alcohol abuse in domestic violence). Alcohol abusers may also alienate friends, relatives, or others. Alcohol abuse may also accompany other unhealthy behaviors such as smoking or the use of illicit drugs. For this particular survey question, only respondents who reported having had at least one drink in the past 12 months are included.

According to this survey, the most typical problem reported by persons aged 25 years and younger within the past year was with tossing down drinks quickly to get the effect. The most common problem reported by those aged 26 years and older was with drinking alone. Adolescents who reported having had at least one drink within the past year frequently reported taking a quick drink when no one was looking—more than the other age groups—possibly to avoid detection for being under the legal drinking age.

Source U.S. Department of Justice. Office of Justice Programs. Bureau of Justice Statistics. *Sourcebook of Criminal Justice Statistics—1992,* Kathleen Maguire, Ann L. Pastore, and Timothy J. Flanagan, eds. Washington, D.C.: U. S. Government Printing Office, [1993], table 3.105, p. 346. Primary source: U.S. Department of Health and Human Services, Substance Abuse and Mental Health Services Administration, *National Household Survey on Drug Abuse: Highlights 1991*, p. 128.

Contact U.S. Department of Health and Human Services, Alcohol, Drug Abuse, and Mental Health Administration, National Institute on Drug Abuse, 5600 Fishers Lane, Rockville, MD 20857; (301) 443-6487. Public Relations: (301) 443-1124. National Clearinghouse for Alcohol and Drug Information: (800) 729-6686.

Consumption of Alcohol by Age Group: 1974–91

Estimated use of alcohol by three age groups, given as percent of each reporting
if they have ever consumed alcohol.

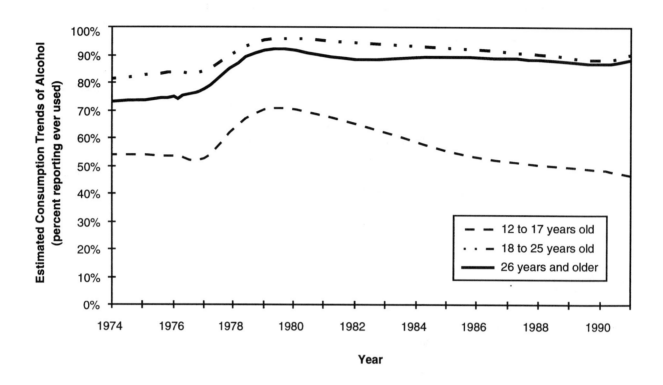

Year	12 to 17 Years Old	18 to 25 Years Old	26 Years and Older
1974	54.0	81.6	73.2
1976	53.6	83.6	74.7
1977	52.6	84.2	77.9
1979	70.3	95.3	91.5
1982	65.2	94.6	88.2
1985	55.5	92.6	89.4
1988	50.2	90.3	88.6
1990	48.2	88.2	86.8
1991	46.4	90.2	88.6

Comments

The National Survey on Drug Abuse is administered by the National Institute on Drug Abuse in a series of surveys measuring the prevalence of drug use in the United States. In 1991, the survey measured the prevalence of drug use among a sample of 32,594 individuals from the civilian, noninstitutionalized population of the U.S. For the first time this survey included Alaska and Hawaii, as well as individuals living in group quarters (e.g., civilians on military installations, individuals living in college dormitories, or individuals living in homeless shelters).

For the years listed on the graph not included in the data table (1975, 1978, 1980, 1981, 1983, 1984, 1986, 1987, and 1989), the values have been *interpolated*. This means that the values for the unknown years were estimated and inserted between the values of two known years. This method of estimation can be useful but may be inaccurate if the value for an unknown is unusually high or low.

According to these statistics, the proportion of individuals who have ever consumed alcohol is much greater for the older groups than for the adolescent group. This should come as no surprise, since the legal drinking age ranged from 18–21 (depending on the particular state) during the mid-1970s and 1980s. As of 1993, the legal drinking age was 21 in all states and 18 in Puerto Rico. This means that those in the youngest group who have consumed alcohol have done so illegally.

Among all groups, abstinence from alcohol declined in the late 1970s to early 1980s. Since the mid-1980s, the prevalence of alcohol use among adolescents has decreased, while the use of alcohol by the adult groups has only declined mildly.

One reason the youth statistics may show more fluctuation is that an individual's response cannot go back and forth between the categories over time. For instance, consider the individual who tries an alcoholic beverage once. His or her reply to the question of whether or not they have ever had an alcoholic drink can never be changed back to a "no." Therefore, because of this one-way progression, the "no" category will shrink over time and will only grow if replaced by youths who have never consumed alcohol.

Source

U.S. Department of Justice. Office of Justice Programs. Bureau of Justice Statistics. *Sourcebook of Criminal Justice Statistics—1992,* Kathleen Maguire, Ann L. Pastore, and Timothy J. Flanagan, eds. Washington, D.C.: U. S. Government Printing Office, [1993], p. 336. Primary source: U.S. Department of Health and Human Services, Substance Abuse and Mental Health Services Administration, *National Household Survey on Drug Abuse: Highlights 1991*, pp. 73, 76, 79.

Contact

U.S. Department of Health and Human Services, Alcohol, Drug Abuse, and Mental Health Administration, National Institute on Drug Abuse, 5600 Fishers Lane, Rockville, MD 20857; (301) 443-6487. Public Relations: (301) 443-1124. National Clearinghouse for Alcohol and Drug Information: (800)729-6686.

Demographic Characteristics of Alcohol Users: 1991

Characteristics of alcohol consumers classified by percentage using alcohol within certain time frames.

N=32,594	Never Used	Ever Used	Used Within Last Year	Used Within Last 30 Days
Total	15.4%	84.6%	68.0%	50.9%
Gender				
Male	11.0	89.0	72.7	58.1
Female	19.4	80.6	63.8	44.3
Race, ethnicity				
White	13.3	86.7	69.9	52.7
Black	21.0	79.0	59.7	43.7
Hispanic	22.6	77.4	64.9	47.5
Age				
12 – 17 years	53.6	46.4	40.3	20.3
18– 25 years	9.8	90.2	82.8	63.6
26 –34 years	7.6	92.4	80.9	61.7
35 years and older	12.6	87.4	64.9	49.5
Population density				
Large metro	13.8	86.2	72.1	55.7
Small metro	14.6	85.4	68.7	51.8
Nonmetro	19.3	80.7	59.7	40.8
Region				
Northeast	13.3	86.7	73.7	56.3
North Central	12.5	87.5	71.9	52.3
South	19.6	80.4	60.1	44.0
West	13.2	86.8	72.2	56.3
Adult education*				
Less than high school	18.9	81.1	54.8	39.8
High school graduate	11.6	88.4	71.2	53.1
Some college	7.6	92.4	77.5	59.1
College graduate	6.0	94.0	81.3	66.1
Current employment†				
Full-time	7.3	92.7	78.4	61.9
Part-time	10.2	89.8	75.7	56.1
Unemployed	10.6	89.4	75.0	58.1
Other‡	18.2	81.8	56.0	39.6

* Data on adult education are not applicable for 12 to 17 year olds. Percents are based on those 18 and older (N=24,589).
† Data on current employment are not applicable for 12 to 17 year olds. Percents are based on those 18 years and older.
‡ Retired, disabled, homemaker, student, or "other."

Comments Alcohol consumption varies widely among individuals, as is apparent by the data shown here. Some 32,594 persons were surveyed through random samplings from all households in the nation by the National Institute on Drug Abuse in order to measure the prevalence of alcohol use in the United States.

According to the statistics presented by the survey, persons most likely to have consumed alcohol within the past 30 days included: males, whites, persons aged 18 to 25 years, large metropolitan area dwellers, residents of the Northeast, college graduates, and full-time employees. These observations do not necessarily lead to the conclusion that an individual matching all these descriptions will have used alcohol within the past 30 days. If, however, one were to sample any group of people who most recently used alcohol within the past 30 days, the chances of finding a person matching that description would be greater than any other combination of characteristics, since each characteristic represents the greatest percentage under the category "used within last 30 days."

Source U.S. Department of Justice. Office of Justice Programs. Bureau of Justice Statistics. *Sourcebook of Criminal Justice Statistics—1992,* Kathleen Maguire, Ann L. Pastore, and Timothy J. Flanagan, eds. Washington, D.C.: U. S. Government Printing Office, [1993], table 3.105, p. 346. Primary source: U.S. Department of Health and Human Services, Substance Abuse and Mental Health Services Administration, *National Household Survey on Drug Abuse: Highlights 1991*, pp. 42–44, 55–57, 91–93.

Contact U.S. Department of Health and Human Services, Alcohol, Drug Abuse, and Mental Health Administration, National Institute on Drug Abuse, 5600 Fishers Lane, Rockville, MD 20857; (301) 443-6487. Public Relations: (301) 443-1124. National Clearinghouse for Alcohol and Drug Information: (800)729-6686.

Past Month Alcohol Use:1974–91

Percent of respondents using alcohol in the month previous to survey, according to age group.

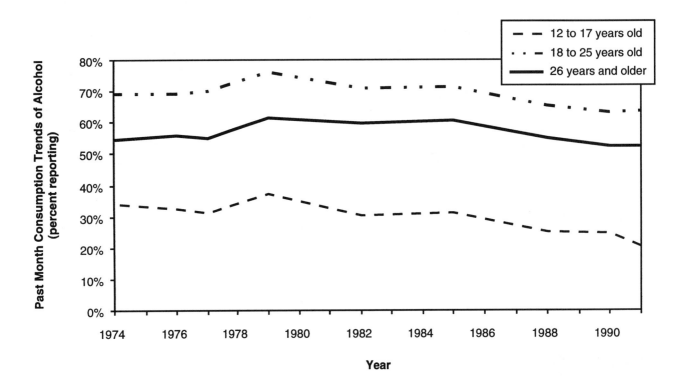

Year	12–17 Yrs.	18–25 Yrs.	26 Yrs. and Older
1974	34.0	69.3	54.5
1976	32.4	69.0	56.0
1977	31.2	70.0	54.9
1979	37.2	75.9	61.3
1982	30.2	70.9	59.8
1985	31.0	71.4	60.6
1988	25.2	65.3	54.8
1990	24.5	63.3	52.3
1991	20.3	63.6	52.5

Comments According to this graph, persons between the ages of 18 and 25 years are more likely to have consumed alcoholic beverages within the past month than persons of younger or older ages. For the years shown on the graph with no data (1975, 1978, 1980, 1981, 1983, 1984, 1986, 1987, and 1989), consumption was estimated between the known values of two other years.

The majority of respondents aged 18 and older had consumed alcohol within the past month for each year during the period of analysis. Consumption trends for all three groups show a decline from 1974–91. The greatest percentage decline was among persons aged 12 to 17 years.

Consumption among adolescents, as shown by this trend, may perhaps be influenced by drinking trends among older groups, although it has started to show some independent decline since 1990.

Source U.S. Department of Justice. Office of Justice Programs. Bureau of Justice Statistics. *Sourcebook of Criminal Justice Statistics—1992,* Kathleen Maguire, Ann L. Pastore, and Timothy J. Flanagan, eds. Washington, D.C.: U. S. Government Printing Office, [1993], table 3.105, p. 346. Primary source: U.S. Department of Health and Human Services, Substance Abuse and Mental Health Services Administration, *National Household Survey on Drug Abuse: Highlights 1991,* pp. 75, 78, 81.

Contact U.S. Department of Health and Human Services, Alcohol, Drug Abuse, and Mental Health Administration, National Institute on Drug Abuse, 5600 Fishers Lane, Rockville, MD 20857: (301) 443-6487. Public Relations: (301) 443-1124. National Clearinghouse for Alcohol and Drug Information: (800)729-6686.

Alcohol Use by High School Seniors: 1982–93

Patterns of alcohol use among high school seniors, according to percent responding.

Year	5+ Drinks in Past Two Weeks	Past Month	Past Year	Ever Used
1975	36.8	68.2	84.8	90.4
1976	37.1	68.3	85.7	91.9
1977	39.4	71.2	87.0	92.5
1978	40.3	72.1	87.7	93.1
1979	41.2	71.8	88.1	93.0
1980	41.2	72.0	87.9	93.2
1981	41.4	70.7	87.0	92.6
1982	40.5	69.7	86.8	92.8
1983	40.8	69.4	87.3	92.6
1984	38.7	67.2	86.0	92.6
1985	36.7	65.9	85.6	92.2
1986	36.8	65.3	84.5	91.3
1987	37.5	66.4	85.7	92.2
1988	34.7	63.9	85.3	92.0
1989	33.0	60.0	82.7	90.7
1990	32.2	57.1	80.6	89.5
1991	29.8	54.0	77.7	88.0
1992	27.9	51.3	76.8	87.5
1993	27.5	51.0	76.0	87.0

Comments Each year since 1975, alcohol use among high school seniors has been reported by a survey conducted by the University of Michigan's Institute for Social Research, as funded by the National Institute on Drug Abuse. About 16,000 seniors from 139 public and private schools nationwide were surveyed in the spring of 1994. After 1993, the wording of the questionnaire was changed so that the responses regarding alcohol consumption for 1994 would not be comparable to previous years.

According to the chart, the proportion of high school seniors who had ever used alcohol fell from a peak of 93.2% in 1980 to 87.0% in 1993. Alcohol use within the past twelve months among seniors peaked in 1979 at 88.1% and steadily decreased to a low of 76.0% in 1993. The proportion of seniors who had used alcohol within the past months reached its zenith in 1978, at 72.1%. The percentage of seniors having consumed five or more alcoholic beverages within the last two weeks was at its highest in 1981, at 41.4%. The similarities among these patterns, all peaking between 1978–81, indicate that alcohol use among high school seniors was most common during those years.

Source U.S. Department of Transportation. National Highway Traffic Safety Administration. Alcohol and State Programs. *Youth Fatal Crash and Alcohol Facts 1993.* U. S Department of Health and Human Services. Public Health Service. Substance Abuse and Mental Health Services Administration. National Institute on Drug Abuse. *Monitoring the Future Study, 1975–1994: National High School Senior Drug Abuse Survey,* 1994.

Contact U.S. Department of Transportation, National Highway Traffic Safety Administration, Alcohol and State Programs, 400 7th St. SW, Washington, D.C. 20590. Office of Public and Consumer Affairs: (202)366-9550. U.S. Department of Health and Human Services, Alcohol, Drug Abuse, and Mental Health Administration, National Institute on Drug Abuse, 5600 Fishers Lane, Rockville, MD 20857; (301) 443-6487. Public Relations: (301) 443-1124. National Clearinghouse for Alcohol and Drug Information: (800) 729-6686.

Drinking and Other Unhealthy Behaviors in Adolescents: 1992

Percent of respondents aged 14–21 who reported drinking alcohol and engaging in other unhealthy behaviors, according to gender.

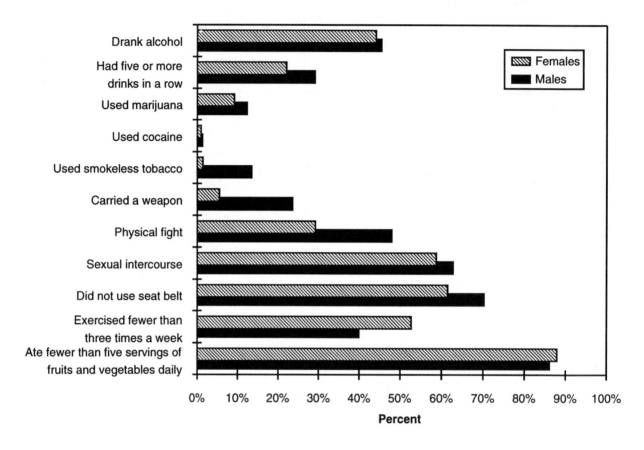

Selected Unhealthy Behavior	Males	Females
Drank alcohol	45.3%	44.0%
Had five or more drinks in a row	29.1%	22.0%
Used marijuana	12.2%	9.2%
Used cocaine	1.4%	1.0%
Used smokeless tobacco	13.4%	1.5%
Carried a weapon	23.5%	5.6%
Physical fight	47.9%	29.2%
Sexual intercourse[1]	62.7%	58.7%
Did not use seat belt	70.2%	61.4%
Exercised fewer than three times a week	39.9%	52.7%
Ate fewer than five servings of fruits and vegetables daily	86.1%	87.9%

[1] Ages 14–21 years and never married.

Comments A recent Surgeon General's Report ("Preventing Tobacco Use Among Young People," 1994) showed the relationship between drinking and other health-threatening behaviors, such as using illicit drugs, smoking cigarettes, carrying weapons, engaging in physical fights, ever having had sexual intercourse, failure to wear seat belts, lack of exercise, and eating less than five servings of fruits and vegetables per day.

Alcohol consumption among youths has serious short-term and long-term health consequences. According to these estimates from the National Health Interview Survey of Youth Risk Behavior, there was little difference between males and females in the percentages of adolescents who had engaged in drinking alcohol within the past 30 days (45.3% for males, 44.0% for females). Males, however, were a little more likely than females to have had more than five drinks in a row within the past 30 days (29.1% for males, 22.0% for females).

Source U.S. Department of Health and Human Services. Public Health Service. Centers for Disease Control and Prevention. National Center for Health Statistics. "Relationship Between Cigarette Smoking and Other Unhealthy Behaviors Among our Nation's Youth: United States, 1992," by J.C. Willard and C.A. Schoenborn, *Advance Data from Vital and Health Statistics No. 263.* Washington, D.C.: U. S. Government Printing Office, 1995.

Contact U. S. Department of Health and Human Services, Public Health Service, Centers for Disease Control and Prevention, National Center for Health Statistics, 6525 Belcrest Rd., Hyattsville, MD 29782; (301) 436-8500.

Adolescent Drinking and Smoking: 1992

Percent of youths aged 12–21 who drank alcohol in the month previous to survey,
compared by gender and by smoking status.

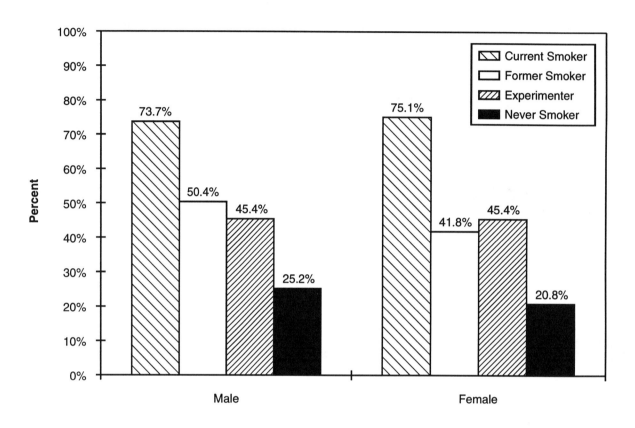

Smoking Status	Male	Female
Current smoker	73.7%	75.1%
Former smoker	50.4%	41.8%
Experimenter	45.4%	45.4%
Never smoker	25.2%	20.8%

Comments   A recent Surgeon General's Report ("Preventing Tobacco Use Among Young People," 1994) showed the relationship between drinking, and other health-threatening behaviors such as using illicit drugs, smoking cigarettes or using smokeless tobacco products, carrying weapons, engaging in physical fights, ever having had sexual intercourse, failure to wear seat belts, lack of exercise, and eating less than five servings of fruits and vegetables per day. Consumption of alcohol among youths may also accompany other risky behaviors, such as smoking.

According to further findings in this report by the National Center for Health Statistics, about three-quarters (74.4%) of current smokers aged 12–21 years old had consumed alcohol in the past 30 days, compared with just 23.0% of those who had never smoked. Of those youths who drank alcohol within the past 30 days, the proportion of current female smokers slightly exceeded current male smokers (75.1% female, 73.7% male), but the percentage of male former smokers was higher than female former smokers (50.4% male, 41.8% female). Adolescents who had consumed alcohol within the past 30 days and were experimenter smokers (youths who have tried cigarettes but have never smoked every day for 30 days and had not used cigarettes in the past 30 days), were equally likely to be male or female.

Source   U.S. Department of Health and Human Services. Public Health Service. Centers for Disease Control and Prevention. National Center for Health Statistics. "Relationship Between Cigarette Smoking and Other Unhealthy Behaviors Among our Nation's Youth: United States, 1992," by J.C. Willard and C.A. Schoenborn, *Advance Data from Vital and Health Statistics No. 263.* Washington, D.C.: U. S. Government Printing Office, 1995.

Contact   U. S. Department of Health and Human Services, Public Health Service, Centers for Disease Control and Prevention, National Center for Health Statistics, 6525 Belcrest Rd., Hyattsville, MD 29782; (301) 436-8500.

Fatal Traffic Injuries Involving Alcohol: 1983–93

Proportions of all fatally injured drivers and pedestrians who were severely impaired by alcohol (drunk).

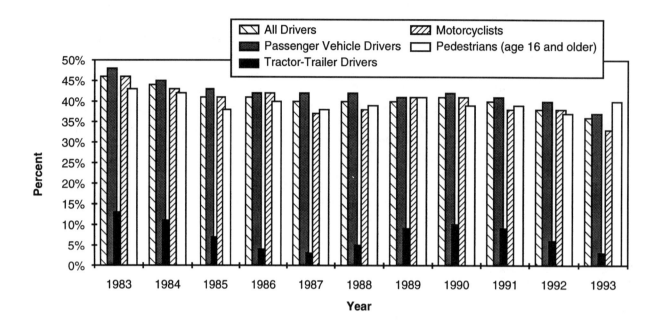

Year	All Drivers	Passenger Vehicle Drivers	Tractor-Trailer Drivers	Motorcyclists	Pedestrians (age 16 and older)
1983	46%	48%	13%	46%	43%
1984	44%	45%	11%	43%	42%
1985	41%	43%	7%	41%	38%
1986	41%	42%	4%	42%	40%
1987	40%	42%	3%	37%	38%
1988	40%	42%	5%	38%	39%
1989	40%	41%	9%	41%	41%
1990	41%	42%	10%	41%	39%
1991	40%	41%	9%	38%	39%
1992	38%	40%	6%	38%	37%
1993	36%	37%	3%	33%	40%

Comments Driving under the influence of alcohol impairs judgment and reflexes. An inebriated driver not only risks personal safety, but is a potential threat to the safety of others on the road. Alcohol impairment is often measured through blood alcohol concentrations (BACs). BAC is the measure of the amount of alcohol in a person's blood, given in grams per deciliter (g/dL, with 100 grams = one deciliter). A BAC of 0.05-0.09 usually indicates moderate alcohol impairment, while an individual with a BAC of 0.10 or higher is considered legally drunk in many states. The percentages shown here are only for those persons with a BAC of 0.10 or higher.

Although the percentages give no indication of the actual number of drunk drivers killed on the road, the overall trend from 1983–93 has been a decrease in the proportion of fatally injured drunk drivers. This does not necessarily mean that fewer people are drinking and driving, only that proportionally fewer of the drivers who are fatally injured each year happen to be drunk. The proportions of fatally injured passenger vehicle drivers have followed the overall trend by gradually declining during 1983–93. Fatal injuries involving tractor-trailer drivers, however, have decreased overall but have fluctuated more widely from year to year. One possible explanation for the fluctuation among tractor-trailer drivers is the fact that there are fewer of them than passenger vehicle drivers. One fatality among tractor-trailer drivers makes a bigger impact on the statistics, which is a percent.

Although the percentage of fatally injured drivers severely impaired by alcohol has decreased, the proportion of drunk pedestrians killed in accidents has remained more stable during the period shown here.

Source Insurance Institute for Highway Safety. "Alcohol," *Fatality Facts 1994,* July 1994.

Contact Insurance Institute for Highway Safety, 1005 North Glebe Rd., Arlington, VA 22201; (703) 247-1500.

Motor Vehicle Crash Fatalities by State: 1993

For each state, the number of auto crash fatalities involving alcohol and the corresponding percent
of all auto crash fatalities, according to the blood alcohol concentration (*BAC), 1993.
Also the percentage point difference in the proportion of alcohol-involved fatalities, 1982–93.

State	*BAC = 0.00 g/dL		*BAC = 0.01–0.09 g/dL		*BAC > 0.10 g/dL		Total Fatalities	Percent Change from 1982 to 1993
	No.	%	No.	%	No.	%		
Alabama	595	57.1	71	6.9	379	36.1	1,042	−12.8
Alaska	68	57.6	3	2.2	47	40.2	118	−12.4
Arizona	401	50.1	68	8.5	332	41.4	801	−6.4
Arkansas	317	54.4	57	9.8	209	35.8	583	−15.4
California	2,403	57.7	406	9.8	1,354	32.5	4,163	−16.7
Colorado	329	58.8	31	5.5	200	35.7	559	−21.1
Connecticut	192	56.2	23	6.8	126	37.0	342	−24.5
Delaware	57	51.7	9	7.9	45	40.4	111	−17.6
District of Columbia	32	56.8	7	12.3	18	30.9	57	−16.5
Florida	1,468	55.7	203	7.7	964	36.6	2,635	−2.3
Georgia	839	60.2	129	9.2	426	30.6	1,394	−18.8
Hawaii	59	44.3	19	14.2	56	41.6	134	−5.6
Idaho	114	50.3	21	9.4	91	40.3	227	+5.7
Illinois	763	54.8	118	8.5	511	36.7	1,392	−13.4
Indiana	556	62.5	75	8.4	258	29.1	889	−11.0
Iowa	255	55.6	50	10.8	154	33.6	459	−2.6
Kansas	280	65.4	31	7.2	117	27.4	428	−10.5
Kentucky	550	63.2	67	7.7	254	29.2	871	−17.0
Louisiana	396	45.1	113	12.8	370	42.1	879	+0.4
Maine	110	59.5	16	8.7	59	31.8	185	−9.1
Maryland	477	71.8	48	7.2	140	21.0	665	−26.2
Massachusetts	258	54.4	52	10.9	165	34.7	475	−13.9
Michigan	792	56.3	122	8.7	493	35.0	1,408	−15.9
Minnesota	326	60.5	42	7.7	171	31.7	538	−15.1
Mississippi	427	52.5	82	10.0	304	37.4	813	−8.9
Missouri	454	47.9	101	10.7	392	41.4	947	+2.0
Montana	81	41.5	18	9.3	96	49.2	195	−7.3
Nebraska	147	57.9	36	14.3	71	27.9	254	−5.8
Nevada	135	51.3	31	11.9	97	36.9	263	−18.0
New Hampshire	74	60.9	9	7.6	38	31.5	121	−19.3
New Jersey	501	63.6	76	9.6	211	26.7	788	−19.7
New Mexico	179	41.6	44	10.3	207	48.1	431	−5.2
New York	1,186	66.6	146	8.2	449	25.2	1,781	−13.7

*BAC is the measure of the amount of alcohol in a person's blood, given in grams per deciliter (g/dL, with 100 grams = one deciliter).

[Continued]

Motor Vehicle Crash Fatalities by State: 1993

[Continued]

State	*BAC = 0.00 g/dL		*BAC = 0.01–0.09 g/dL		*BAC > 0.10 g/dL		Total Fatalities	Percent Change from 1982 to 1993
	No.	%	No.	%	No.	%		
North Carolina	875	63.0	97	7.0	417	30.0	1,389	−23.1
North Dakota	44	48.9	5	5.6	40	45.5	89	−13.0
Ohio	959	64.7	107	7.2	416	28.1	1,482	−21.2
Oklahoma	402	59.8	57	8.5	213	31.7	671	−15.9
Oregon	307	58.6	54	10.2	164	31.2	524	−21.4
Pennsylvania	842	55.1	110	7.2	577	37.8	1,529	−13.4
Rhode Island	35	46.9	8	11.0	31	42.1	74	−13.1
South Carolina	610	72.1	37	4.4	199	23.5	846	−31.0
South Dakota	81	57.6	7	5.1	52	37.3	140	−17.8
Tennessee	649	55.4	101	8.6	422	36.0	1,171	−17.8
Texas	1,248	41.1	325	10.7	1,464	48.2	3,037	−9.6
Utah	206	67.9	21	7.0	76	25.1	303	−6.1
Vermont	61	55.8	9	8.4	39	35.8	110	−20.1
Virginia	481	54.8	87	9.9	310	35.3	878	−7.6
Washington	327	49.5	47	7.1	287	43.4	661	−12.9
West Virginia	245	57.0	23	5.3	161	37.6	429	−7.9
Wisconsin	392	54.9	54	7.6	268	37.5	714	−16.5
Wyoming	69	57.5	6	4.6	45	37.9	120	−12.9

*BAC is the measure of the amount of alcohol in a person's blood, given in grams per deciliter (g/dL, with 100 grams = one deciliter).

Comments

Alcohol involvement in traffic fatalities from state to state is related to a variety of factors, including population characteristics, urbanization, and vehicle mix. In addition, the accuracy of estimates for each state depends entirely upon the proportion of drivers, pedestrians, and bicyclists in fatal crashes for whom a blood alcohol concentration (BAC) test result is known.

During 1993, test results were known for 45% of active reporting agencies nationwide regarding fatal crashes, but ranged from 12–83% for the 50 states and the District of Columbia. Since reporting conditions varied significantly between states, these factors make direct state-to-state comparisons unreliable.

Source

U.S. Department of Health and Human Services. Public Health Service. Centers for Disease Control and Prevention. "Update: Alcohol-Related Traffic Fatalities, 1982–1993." *Morbidity and Mortality Weekly Report* 43, No. 47 (1994): pp. 861–865. Primary source: Fatal Accident Reporting System, U.S. Department of Transporatation.

Contact

U.S. Department of Transportation, National Highway Traffic Safety Administration, 400 7th St. SW, Washington, D.C. 20590. Office of Public and Consumer Affairs: (202) 366-9550.

Blood Alcohol Concentrations (BACs) of Fatally Injured Drivers: 1993

Percent of passenger vehicle drivers who had blood alcohol concentrations (*BACs)
at or exceeding 0.10%, according to age group and gender.

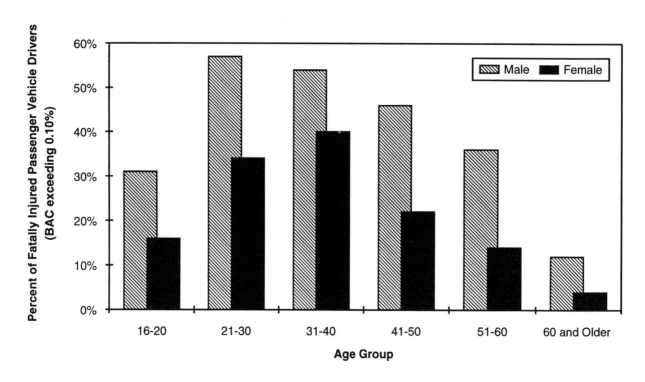

Age	Male	Female	Total
16–20	31%	16%	27%
21–30	57%	34%	51%
31–40	54%	40%	50%
41–50	46%	22%	39%
51–60	36%	14%	29%
60 and older	12%	4%	9%
TOTAL	42%	23%	37%

*BAC is the measure of the amount of alcohol in a person's blood, given in grams per
deciliter (g/dL, with 100 grams = one deciliter).

Comments Persons who drive while impaired by drugs or alcohol are a hazard to themselves and others. Each year, alcohol-related motor vehicle crashes kill approximately 17,500 persons in the United States. Impaired driving is a leading cause of death among persons under 25 years of age.

In 1993, some 37% of all drivers who were fatally injured in passenger vehicle accidents were considered legally drunk, but the frequency of drunk drivers varied greatly by age and gender. A fatally injured driver who was legally drunk at the time of the crash in 1993 was more likely to be male than female, and more likely to be between the ages of 21 and 30, according to these Department of Transportation statistics. Among women, however, most fatally injured drunk drivers were in their 30s.

Source U.S. Department of Health and Human Services. Public Health Service. Centers for Disease Control and Prevention. "Update: Alcohol-Related Traffic Fatalities, 1982–1993." *Morbidity and Mortality Weekly Report* 43, No. 47 (1994): pp. 861–865. Primary source: Fatal Accident Reporting System, U.S. Department of Transporatation.

Contact U.S. Department of Transportation, National Highway Traffic Safety Administration, 400 7th St. SW, Washington, D.C. 20590. Office of Public and Consumer Affairs: (202) 366-9550.

Fatalities in Alcohol-Related Traffic Accidents: 1982–91

Estimated U.S. fatalities in motor vehicle accidents,
according to blood alcohol concentrations (*BACs).

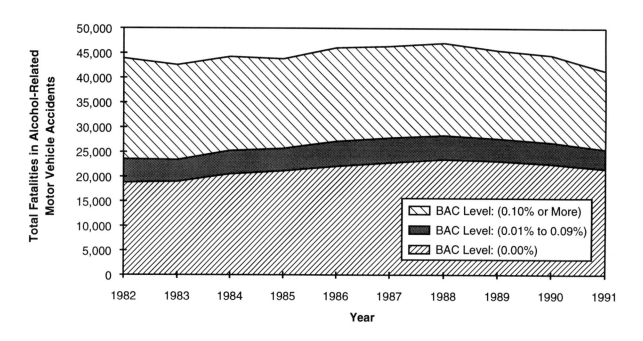

Year	Total Fatalities	Total Fatalities in Crashes	*BAC Level: No Alcohol (0.00%)	*BAC Level: Some and Impaired (0.01 to 0.09%)	*BAC Level: Intoxicated (0.10% or more)
1982	43,945	25,165	18,780	4,809	20,356
1983	42,589	23,646	18,943	4,472	19,174
1984	44,257	23,758	20,499	4,766	18,992
1985	43,825	22,715	21,109	4,604	18,111
1986	46,087	24,045	22,042	5,109	18,936
1987	46,390	23,641	22,749	5,112	18,529
1988	47,087	23,626	23,461	4,895	18,731
1989	45,582	22,436	23,146	4,574	17,862
1990	44,599	22,084	22,515	4,434	17,650
1991	41,462	19,900	21,563	3,956	15,944

*BAC is the measure of the amount of alcohol in a person's blood, given in grams per deciliter (g/dL, with 100 grams = one deciliter).

Comments

Each year the National Highway Traffic Safety Administration (part of the U.S. Department of Transportation) collects data based on information submitted by all 50 states, the District of Columbia, and Puerto Rico. From this data national statistics are derived on blood alcohol levels of motor vehicle drivers involved in fatal accidents. The probability of alcohol involvement of each driver for whom there is no BAC data is calculated based on known test results for people in similar accidents using specific driver and crash parameters. This procedure allows national estimates of alcohol-related motor vehicle fatalities to be derived.

According to these statistics, the frequency of no alcohol involvement in fatal crashes has risen since early 1980s, and the frequency of intoxicated drivers involved in fatal crashes has decreased. However, the relative frequency of drivers with some alcohol impairment (but not legally intoxicated) who were involved in fatal crashes has remained fairly steady, varying only between 9.5–11.1% during the ten years examined.

These trends may reflect a change in public attitudes regarding drinking and driving especially toward drunk drivers. The stable rate of alcohol-impaired drivers involved in fatal crashes may indicate an unwillingness among some to totally abstain from driving when drinking alcohol.

Source

U.S. Department of Justice. Office of Justice Programs. Bureau of Justice Statistics. *Sourcebook of Criminal Justice Statistics—1992,* Kathleen Maguire, Ann L. Pastore, and Timothy J. Flanagan, eds. Washington, D.C.: U. S. Government Printing Office, [1993], p. 355. Primary source: U.S. Department of Transportation, National Highway Traffic Safety Administration, *Fatal Accident Reporting System, 1991*, p. 38.

Contact

U.S. Department of Transportation, National Highway Traffic Safety Administration, 400 7th St. SW, Washington, D.C. 20590. Office of Public and Consumer Affairs: (202) 366-9550.

Alcohol Involvement in Automobile Crashes: 1988–91

Auto crash comparisons in relation to severity and percent of each involving alcohol.

Year	Total	Alcohol Involvement	Percent Alcohol Involvement
Total Crashes			
1988	6,877,000	479,000	7%
1989	6,664,000	398,000	6%
1990	6,462,000	469,000	7%
1991	6,110,000	491,000	8%
Crash Severity: Property Damage Only			
1988	4,633,000	226,000	5%
1989	4,450,000	181,000	4%
1990	4,255,000	220,000	5%
1991	4,073,000	259,000	6%
Crash Severity: Minor or Moderate Injury			
1988	1,828,000	177,000	10%
1989	1,800,000	148,000	8%
1990	1,825,000	173,000	9%
1991	1,681,000	165,000	10%
Crash Severity: Severe or Fatal Injury			
1988	415,000	76,000	18%
1989	394,000	68,000	17%
1990	382,000	77,000	20%
1991	357,000	68,000	19%

Comments The data presented here are from annual reports of overall crash statistics produced from information collected by the General Estimates System (GES) for the National Highway Traffic Safety Administration (NHTSA). The GES obtained its data from a nationally representative probability sample selected from an estimated 6.9 million police-reported traffic crashes in 1988; about 6.6 million in 1989; approximately 6.5 million in 1990; and 6.1 million in 1991.

The corresponding GES sample of police accident reports drawn was 49,000 in 1988; 44,000 in 1989; 46,000 in 1990; and 42,600 in 1991. These data came from approximately 400 police agencies within 60 geographic sites across the U.S. (The variety of sites leads to sampling variation.) Alcohol involvement was mentioned by police officers only when evidence of alcohol was present. This does not necessarily mean that a driver, passenger, or nonoccupant was tested for evidence of alcohol consumption.

Within the four years covered by these statistics, the frequency of alcohol involvement increased as the severity of the crash increased. This relationship implies that when alcohol is involved in an automobile crash, it is likely to be more severe than if no alcohol were involved. For example, although alcohol was only involved in 8% of all crashes in 1991, it was involved in 19% of all severe or fatal crashes that year.

Source U.S. Department of Justice. Office of Justice Programs. Bureau of Justice Statistics. *Sourcebook of Criminal Justice Statistics—1992,* Kathleen Maguire, Ann L. Pastore, and Timothy J. Flanagan, eds. Washington, D.C.: U. S. Government Printing Office, [1993], p. 356. U.S. Primary source: U.S. Department of Transportation, National Highway Traffic Safety Administration, *General Estimates System 1988*, p. 38; *1989*, p. 38; *1990*, p. 44; *1991*, p. 50.

Contact U.S. Department of Transportation, National Highway Traffic Safety Administration, 400 7th St. SW, Washington, D.C. 20590. Office of Public and Consumer Affairs: (202) 366-9550.

Lives Saved by Drinking Age Laws and Alcohol-Related Youth Fatalities, 1985–93

The cumulative estimated number of lives saved by minimum drinking age laws,
and the cumulative number of alcohol-related youth fatalities, starting from a baseline of 1984.

Cumulative Lives Saved and Cumulative Alcohol Fatalities, Baseline 1984

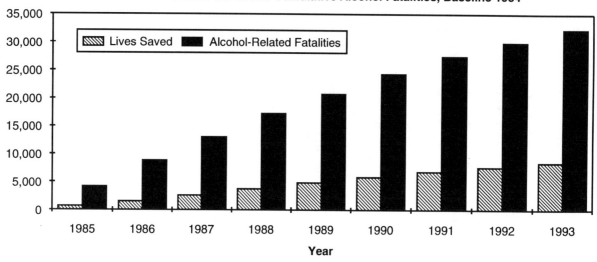

Year	Cumulative Lives Saved, Baseline 1975	Cumulative Lives Saved, Baseline 1984	Cumulative Alcohol-Related Youth Fatalities, Baseline 1984
1975-84	5,530	—	—
1985	6,231	701	4,184
1986	7,071	1,541	8,826
1987	8,142	2,612	13,037
1988	9,290	3,760	17,224
1989	10,383	4,853	20,763
1990	11,416	5,886	24,320
1991	12,357	6,827	27,426
1992	13,152	7,622	29,904
1993	13,968	8,438	32,268

Comments   These statistics demonstrate the technique of using a baseline year as a frame of reference. Since the data are measured on a cumulative basis (a running total) it is necessary to establish a point of origin. For the two variables using a baseline of 1984, all entries for the following years are simply summed together, starting from zero in 1984. This does not mean that there were no lives saved or alcohol-related fatalities in 1984, but that the values of those variables for 1984 are being treated as the starting points from which the data for the subsequent years will be added.

For example, by comparing the same variable (cumulative lives saved) for the two baseline years of 1975 and 1984, it is possible to determine how the first value (701) was calculated for the baseline 1984 category. From 1975 to 1984, the estimated number of lives saved by minimum drinking age laws was 5,530, which grew to 6,231 in 1985 (or 701 more than the total at the end of 1984). These statistics attempt to show a relationship between minimum drinking age laws and alcohol-related youth (ages 15-20) fatalities. But it is important to recognize that within the "alcohol-related fatalities," numbers included youths (who may or may not have been drinking) who were hit by older drinking drivers.

Similarly, it is unclear whether or not the values for "lives saved" include only youths or all age groups. As of 1993, all states and the District of Columbia had 21-year-old minimum drinking age laws. By 1994, 29 states and the District of Columbia had set lower blood alcohol levels for youths. Most of these states set a BAC threshold level of 0.02 for all youths under 21.

Source   U.S. Department of Transportation. National Highway Traffic Safety Administration. Alcohol and State Programs. *Youth Fatal Crash and Alcohol Facts, 1993*. Washington, D.C.: U.S. Government Printing Office, [1993].

Contact   U.S. Department of Transportation, National Highway Traffic Safety Administration, 400 7th St. SW, Washington, D.C. 20590. Office of Public and Consumer Affairs: (202) 366-9550.

Fatally Injured Drunk Drivers: 1980–93

Percent of drunk drivers who were killed in auto accidents, according to age group.

Year	16–20	21–30	31 and Over
1980	53%	61%	48%
1981	47%	62%	44%
1982	49%	62%	44%
1983	47%	60%	40%
1984	41%	56%	39%
1985	34%	54%	38%
1986	36%	56%	37%
1987	29%	56%	37%
1988	30%	57%	36%
1989	34%	53%	35%
1990	31%	56%	36%
1991	34%	54%	36%
1992	30%	55%	35%
1993	27%	51%	34%

Comments This chart presents the age distribution of all the passenger vehicle drivers who were severely impaired by alcohol when killed in motor vehicle accidents from 1980 to 1993. A fatally injured driver with severe alcohol impairment is defined here as someone with a blood alcohol concentration equal to or exceeding 0.10%.

According to the chart, the percentage of drunk drivers killed in 1993 dropped for all three age groups from the 1980 levels. However, the groups differed in the amount of change. The proportion drunk drivers killed among the youngest group of drivers (ages 16–20) fell by 26% (from 53% in 1980 to 27% in 1993). The percentage changes from 1980 to 1993 for the two other age groups declined by 10% for those aged 21–30, and 14% for those over 30.

By analyzing these percentages, it *seems* that the youngest drivers as a group became more responsible with alcohol than the other two age groups. It is important to remember, however, that the 16–20 age group has the fewest number of drivers relative to the other groups, since it includes the narrowest age range of only four years. The middle group, aged 21–30, has a broader age range (nine years). The oldest age group, aged 31 and older, is the most inclusive of the three age ranges and represents the majority of those who drive. The smaller the group, the greater the impact upon the group by the actions of a single individual. Likewise, the larger the group, the smaller the impact of one individual's actions. Since the youngest group is likely to have the least total number of drivers, the actions of one individual driver will make a bigger impact on that group than on any other.

Some of the declines for all age groups may genuinely be attributed to an increased social awareness of personal responsibility regarding drinking and driving. An increase in social consideration may have had a greater impact overall upon the youngest and oldest age groups. Other factors, such as increased intolerance of alcohol possession by minors (illegal in most states) and increased penalties for drinking and driving may have also influenced behavior change.

Source Insurance Institute for Highway Safety. "Alcohol," *Fatality Facts 1994,* July 1994.

Contact Insurance Institute for Highway Safety, 1005 North Glebe Rd., Arlington, VA 22201; (703) 247-1500.

Youth Crash Fatalities and Alcohol: 1982–93

Comparison of alcohol vs. non-alcohol related fatalities in auto accidents for youths aged 15–20.

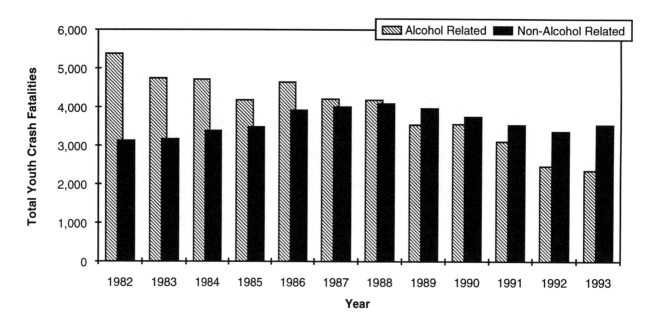

Year	Alcohol Related	Non-Alcohol Related
1982	5,380	3,128
1983	4,747	3,167
1984	4,718	3,383
1985	4,184	3,479
1986	4,642	3,911
1987	4,211	4,002
1988	4,187	4,095
1989	3,539	3,964
1990	3,557	3,751
1991	3,106	3,536
1992	2,478	3,373
1993	2,364	3,541

Comments

The proportions of young (aged 15 through 20) fatally injured drivers and young drivers involved in fatal crashes who were intoxicated have dropped significantly since 1982.

The National Highway Traffic Safety Administration (NHTSA) reported in 1993 that over 40% of all deaths for 15–20 year olds result from motor vehicle crashes, and that two out of five motor vehicle fatalities involve alcohol. By linking these two statistics, one can conclude that if motor vehicle crashes account for a significant portion of youth fatalities and if a significant portion of all motor vehicle fatalities involve alcohol, then a certain proportion of all youth deaths will result from motor vehicle crashes involving alcohol. However, the total number of 15–20 year olds fluctuates from year to year. Therefore, in analyzing the number of crash fatalities, it is not possible to tell how frequent alcohol involvement was for any given year.

The population of the United States aged 15 through 20 declined from 24.2 million in 1982 to 20.8 million in 1993, a drop of 14%. During this period, however, alcohol-related fatalities among that age group decreased by over 56%, which indicates that such a decline was not just caused by a shrinking youth population.

Source

U.S. Department of Transportation. National Highway Traffic Safety Administration. Alcohol and State Programs. *Youth Fatal Crash and Alcohol Facts, 1993*. Washington, D.C.: U.S. Government Printing Office, [1993].

Contact

U.S. Department of Transportation, National Highway Traffic Safety Administration, 400 7th St. SW, Washington, D.C. 20590. Office of Public and Consumer Affairs: (202) 366-9550.

Youth Crash Fatality Rate and Alcohol: 1982–93

Number of persons aged 15–20 killed in motor vehicle crashes
per 100,000 population and the proportion involving alcohol.

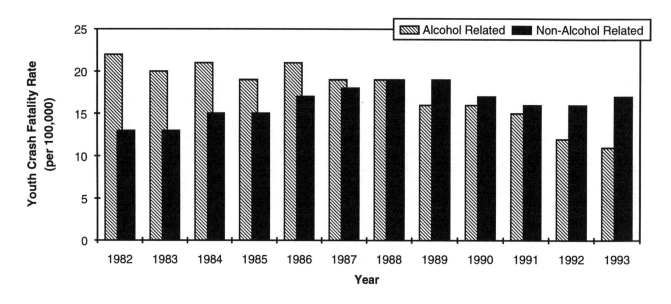

Year	Alcohol Related	Non-Alcohol Related
1982	22	13
1983	20	13
1984	21	15
1985	19	15
1986	21	17
1987	19	18
1988	19	19
1989	16	19
1990	16	17
1991	15	16
1992	12	16
1993	11	17

Comments In the early 1980s, it was more than twice as likely that alcohol was involved when a crash fatality was a youth (aged 15–20). The term "crash fatalities" refers to all those who died in a motor vehicle crash (drivers, passengers, and nonoccupants). An "alcohol-related" fatality is counted if any driver or nonoccupant involved in the crash had been drinking. Therefore, the young person killed may or may not have been drinking.

Throughout the 1980s, the rate of alcohol-related fatalities fell, while the rate for nonalcohol related fatalities climbed steadily. By 1988 the two rates converged and since then, the rate for nonalcohol youth crash fatalities per 100,000 population had exceeded the rate involving alcohol.

Since less than half of the teenage motor vehicle fatalities are alcohol-related, drinking and driving is no longer the leading cause of death for this age group—motor vehicle crashes remain so by far.

These rates, although less specific than the actual numbers of fatalities, are useful in learning about the frequency of alcohol involvement in relation to motor vehicle crashes that kill people aged 15 through 20.

Some of the probable reasons given by the National Highway Traffic Administration to explain the reduction in fatalities from 1982 to 1993 include: minimum age 21 drinking laws, the emergence of a wide range of prevention programs directed at youths, public awareness campaigns, enforcement efforts to prevent underage drinking, and patrolling of places where youths are likely to drink and drive. Also, young persons themselves are increasingly encouraging their peers to avoid the dangers of drinking and impaired driving.

Source U.S. Department of Transportation. National Highway Traffic Safety Administration. Alcohol and State Programs. *Youth*

Fatal Crash and Alcohol Facts, 1993. Washington, D.C.: U.S. Government Printing Office, [1993].

Contact U.S. Department of Transportation, National Highway Traffic Safety Administration, 400 7th St. SW, Washington, D.C.

20590. Office of Public and Consumer Affairs: (202) 366-9550.

DUI Arrests by Demographic Area: 1993

Total DUI (Driving Under the Influence) arrests and DUI arrests of persons
under 18 years of age, by descriptive demographic area, 1993

Area (total population)	Total arrests	Under 18
City (137,365,000)	703,888	6,315
Suburban county (42,794,000)	264,597	1,922
Rural county (20,041,000)	187,713	1,849
Suburban area*	501,480	4,110

Total DUI arrests by gender and descriptive demographic area, 1993

Area	Male	Female	TOTAL
City	600,745	103,143	703,888
Suburban county	230,312	34,285	264,597
Rural county	163,255	24,458	187,713
Suburban area*	429,931	71,549	501,480

Total DUI arrests of persons under 18 years of age
by gender and descriptive demographic area, 1993

Area	Male	Female	TOTAL
City	5,382	943	6,315
Suburban county	1,718	274	1,922
Rural county	1,592	257	1,849
Suburban area*	3,520	590	4,110

* Includes suburban city and county law enforcement agencies within metropolitan areas. Excludes central cities. Suburban cities and counties are also included in other groups.

Comments These statistics reported by the Federal Bureau of Investigation (FBI) show the total number of driving under the influence (DUI) arrests made throughout the United States in 1993. By examining who is arrested and where, it is possible to better understand the problem of drunk driving. According to the FBI, there were 1,229,971 DUI arrests in 1993. City arrests accounted for 753,463 of the total; suburban county arrests, 278,799; rural county arrests, 197,709; and suburban area arrests, 549,668.

The sum of the components just listed exceeds the actual total. This is because the term "suburban area" includes suburban city and county law enforcement agencies within metropolitan areas, so some of the incidents have been counted more than once. Therefore, it is not possible to directly compare "suburban area" with the other three categories. "Suburban area" includes cases also included in the other three categories and does not stand alone. This condition is sometimes referred to as statistical *leakage* or *bleeding*, and can make analysis difficult. It is possible, however, to make some general comparisons between the other three categories. Some cautious general observations may be made using the "suburban areas" category.

In order to make comparisons between the first three categories, one must first create a way to make the information presented in them consistent. To simply state that cities have more DUI arrests than suburban counties (which in turn have more DUI arrests than rural counties) is only superficially relevant. More importantly, someone might want to know how frequently a DUI arrest happens in one of those categories.

By using the total 1993 populations of the three categories analyzed here (total city population = 137,365,000, total suburban county population = 42,794,000, and total rural county population = 20,041,000) it becomes possible to measure the frequency of DUI arrests relative to each region's population. For the category "city," a ratio of 0.5% (703,888 ÷ 137,365,000) indicates that one DUI arrest occurs for about every 200 city residents. Similarly, the DUI ratios for "suburban county" and "rural county" are 0.6% and 0.9%, respectively. These ratios indicate that of the three categories, a DUI arrest per capita occurs most frequently in rural counties, followed by suburban counties, and then in cities. The "suburban area" ratio is 0.6%, but is not comparable to the other three.

It is important to remember, however, that these statistics only measure arrests (supplied by reporting agencies) and do not mention the residence or motive of the arrested driver.

Source U.S. Department of Justice. Federal Bureau of Investigation. *Crime in the United States 1993.* Washington, D.C.: U.S. Government Printing Office, [1994], pp. 220, 238–9, 247–8, 256–7, 265–6.

Contact Federal Bureau of Investigation, Criminal Justice Information Services Division, Programs Support Section, Ninth St. and Pennsylvania Ave. NW, Washington, D.C. 20535. Public Affairs: (202) 324-3691.

Total Arrests for DUI: 1993

Total number of arrests for DUI (Driving Under the Influence), according to age and gender.

	Male	Female	Total
Under 18	9,170	1,552	10,722
Under 10*	90	13	103
10–12	23	10	33
13–14	138	45	183
15	413	100	513
16	2,312	425	2,737
17	6,194	959	7,153
18–24	238,559	34,918	273,477
18	16,273	2,344	18,617
19	22,139	3,149	25,288
20	28,224	3,719	31,943
21	41,018	5,904	46,922
22	44,039	6,661	50,700
23	44,590	6,635	51,225
24	42,276	6,506	48,782
25–29	199,566	33,631	233,197
30–34	196,337	37,154	233,491
35–39	151,640	28,049	179,689
40–44	102,311	17,532	119,843
45–49	65,628	9,971	75,599
50–54	40,132	5,198	45,330
55–59	23,709	2,558	26,267
60–64	14,997	1,435	16,432
65 and older	14,495	1,429	15,924
TOTAL	1,056,544	173,427	1,229,971

* DUI includes operation of mopeds, snowmobiles, boats, tractors, etc.; this may explain how individuals under the legal driving age were arrested for DUI.

Comments Persons who drive vehicles under the influence of alcohol pose a great risk to public safety. When a person drinks and drives, his or her ability to concentrate, judge speed and distance, and react quickly may all be impaired.

A DUI offense involves the operation of any vehicle or common carrier (e.g., cars, trucks, motorcycles, mopeds, snowmobiles, boats, tractors) while under the influence of liquor or narcotics. In 1993, 10,512 law enforcement agencies participated in the survey. These agencies served a population of 214,099,000, and reported 1,229,971 DUI offenses.

In 1993, however, the total U.S. population was estimated at about 258,000,000. Accordingly, the agencies participating in this survey served only 82% of the total U.S. population. Therefore, it is likely that the actual number of DUI offenses in the entire U.S. is higher, and could be as much as 18% higher.

It is temping to use these statistics to compute the percent of Americans arrested for DUI. This would be done by dividing the number of DUI offenses by the total population. However, these statistics report *offenses,* not *individuals.* Accordingly, some individuals may account for multiple offenses. This is the case when an indiviual is arrested two or more times for an alcohol related offense. Therefore, these statistics cannot be used to determine how many individuals are invloved in DUI offenses each year.

Arrests for driving under the influence in 1993 varied greatly by age, with males accounting for the majority of arrests for all age groups. The number of arrests shown here are categorized by age group and gender. Age groups, except for those under 24 years old, cover a five-year span. Since the "18–24" age category represents seven distinct age possibilities instead of five, it is only possible to make general observations for this age groups relative to the others.

Source U.S. Department of Justice. Federal Bureau of Investigation. *Crime in the United* *States 1993.* Washington, D.C.: U.S. Government Printing Office, [1994], pp. 227–232.

Contact U.S. Department of Transportation, National Highway Traffic Safety Administration, 400 7th St. SW, Washington, D.C. 20590. Office of Public and Consumer Affairs: (202) 366-9550. For information concerning the National Uniform Crime Reporting Program: Uniform Crime Reports, Criminal Justice Information Services Division, FBI/GRB, Washington, D.C. 20535. Information Dissemination: (202) 324-5015.

Arrests for Alcohol-Related Offenses and DUI: 1972–93

Number of persons (in thousands) arrested for any alcohol-related offense
compared to number of persons arrested for DUI (Driving Under the Influence).

Year	Alcohol-Related Offenses	Driving Under the Influence
1972	2,835	604
1973	2,539	654
1974	2,297	617
1975	3,044	909
1976	2,790	838
1977	3,303	1,104
1978	3,406	1,205
1979	3,455	1,232
1980	3,535	1,304
1981	3,745	1,422
1982	3,640	1,405
1983	3,729	1,613
1984	3,153	1,347
1985	3,418	1,503
1986	3,325	1,459
1987	3,248	1,410
1988	2,995	1,294
1989	3,180	1,333
1990	3,270	1,391
1991	3,000	1,289
1992	3,061	1,320
1993	2,886	1,230

Comments Arrests for driving under the influence (DUI) make up a portion of all arrests for alcohol-related offenses each year. The FBI classifies arrests for DUI, liquor law violations, drunkenness, disorderly conduct, and vagrancy all as alcohol-related offenses.

Arrests for DUI offenses often comprised over 40% of all arrests for alcohol-related offenses during the 1972–93 period. DUI offenses are often treated more critically by law enforcement agencies than are some of the other alcohol-related offenses. This is because of the serious threat to public safety created by alcohol-impaired drivers.

Although the totals for DUI offenses increased during the period shown here, this increase may not necessarily be caused by more drunk drivers. The number of reporting agencies and the population represented varies from year to year, and complete arrest data were not always available for every state in every year. Such inconsistencies make direct year-to-year comparisons difficult. Furthermore, part of the rise in alcohol-related offenses may be explained by the increase of the total population of licensed drivers in the U.S. since 1972. (During the 1980s alone, the number of licensed drivers increased by over 20 million.)

Source U.S. Department of Justice. Office of Justice Programs. Bureau of Justice Statistics. *Sourcebook of Criminal Justice Statistics—1992,* Kathleen Maguire, Ann L. Pastore, and Timothy J. Flanagan, eds. Washington, D.C.: U. S. Government Printing Office, [1993], table 4.27, p. 456. Primary source: Federal Bureau of Investigation, *Crime in the United States, 1972*, 1973, p. 126; *1973*, p. 128; *1974*, p. 186; *1975*, p. 188; *1976*, p. 181; *1977*, p. 180; *1978*, p. 194; *1979*, p. 196; *1980*, p. 200; *1981*, p. 171; *1982*, pp. 176–77; *1983*, pp. 179–80; *1984*, pp. 172–73; *1985*, pp. 174–75; *1986*, pp. 174–75; *1987*, pp. 174–75; *1988*, pp. 178–79; *1989*, pp. 182–83; *1990*, pp. 184–85; *1991*, pp. 223–24, *1992*, p. 218; *1993*, p. 218.

Contact U.S. Department of Transportation, National Highway Traffic Safety Administration, 400 7th St. SW, Washington, D.C. 20590. Office of Public and Consumer Affairs: (202) 366-9550. For information concerning the National Uniform Crime Reporting Program: Uniform Crime Reports, Criminal Justice Information Services Division, FBI/GRB, Washington, D.C. 20535. Information Dissemination: (202) 324-5015.

Arrests for Drunkenness: 1993

Number of persons arrested for being drunk (excluding DUI), according to age group.

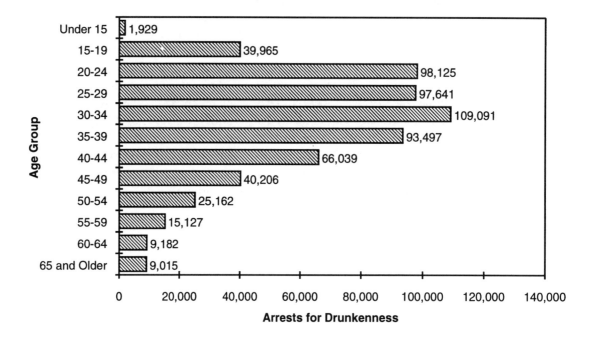

Age Group	Arrestees
Under 15	1,929
15–19	39,965
20–24	98,125
25–29	97,641
30–34	109,091
35–39	93,497
40–44	66,039
45–49	40,206
50–54	25,162
55–59	15,127
60–64	9,182
65 and older	9,015
All ages	604,979

Comments An arrest for drunkenness includes all offenses involving intoxication except for driving under the influence (DUI). An arrest for drunkenness might occur if an individual publicly behaves recklessly or irresponsibly, thereby threatening the safety of others.

The FBI reported that in 1993, the number of arrests for drunkenness totaled 604,979. These figures came from 10,512 reporting agencies, representing a population of 214,099,000.

It should be noted, however, that the total U.S. population in 1993 was estimated at 258,000,000. Consequently, these agencies serve only 82% of the total population of the U.S.

According to these statistics, persons between the ages of 30 and 34 comprised the largest portion of arrestees for drunkenness, followed by the 20–24 age group. This does not necessarily mean that the population of one age group is more inclined to public drunkenness than another, just that there were more people arrested from certain age groups. Some age groups are composed of more individuals than others. Comparisons between specific age groups are misleading since the exact numbers of individuals within the age groups are not given here.

Source U.S. Department of Justice. Federal Bureau of Investigation. *Crime in the United States 1993*. Washington, D.C.: U.S. Government Printing Office, [1994], pp. 227–28.

Contact U.S. Department of Transportation, National Highway Traffic Safety Administration, 400 7th St. SW, Washington, D.C. 20590. Office of Public and Consumer Affairs: (202) 366-9550. For information concerning the National Uniform Crime Reporting Program: Uniform Crime Reports, Criminal Justice Information Services Division, FBI/GRB, Washington, D.C. 20535. Information Dissemination: (202) 324-5015.

Drunkenness Arrests: 1993

The number and rate of arrests for drunkenness in the U.S. according to population group.

Population Group	Number of Reporting Agencies	Population Served	Number of Arrests	Rate (per 100,000 inhabitants)
Rural counties	2,059	22,306,000	40,640	182.2
Suburban counties	1,007	46,243,000	56,860	123.0
Cities, total	7,446	145,549,000	507,479	348.7
Under 10,000 inhabitants	4,917	17,929,000	84,040	468.7
10,000–24,999	1,408	22,238,000	76,276	343.0
25,000–49,999	603	20,982,000	68,849	328.1
50,000–99,999	327	25,502,000	79,873	355.0
100,000–249,999	129	19,156,000	68,398	357.1
250,000 and over	62	42,742,000	130,043	304.2
Suburban area*	5,327	92,137,000	191,630	208.0
Nation, total	10,512	214,099,000	604,979	282.6

* Includes suburban city and county law enforcement agencies within metropolitan areas. Excludes central cities. Suburban cities and counties are also included in other groups.

Comments Arrest practices, policies, and enforcement regarding drunkenness vary from place to place, and even within a community from time to time. (For example, if local police conduct a campaign against another nonviolent crime such as burglary, arrests for drunkenness may drop temporarily.) Also, the definition of drunkenness as applied to an individual who is arrested may be interpreted differently in different areas.

In general, practices for certain unlawful conducts like drunkenness, disorderly conduct, vagrancy, and related violations differ among law enforcement agencies. Practices for robbery, burglary, and other more serious crimes are more likely to be uniform and consistent throughout all jurisdictions.

The arrest figures presented here are only representative of participating law enforcement agencies, and therefore do not necessarily comprise the entire national population for any of the given categories. Also, these arrest figures do not measure the number of individuals arrested, since one person may be arrested several times during the year for drunkenness.

Since each category listed has a different level of participation, the only way to compare the frequency of drunkenness arrests between the categories is to measure the rate of drunkenness arrests (per 100,000 inhabitants) for each. These rates show how often arrests for drunkenness occur within each category. For example, cities with populations under 10,000 had the highest rate of drunkenness arrests (468.7 per 100,000 residents), while cities with populations of 25,000–49,999 had the lowest (328.1 per 100,000 residents).

Source U.S. Department of Justice. Federal Bureau of Investigation. *Crime in the* *United States 1993*. Washington, D.C.: U.S. Government Printing Office, [1994], p. 220.

Contact U.S. Department of Transportation, National Highway Traffic Safety Administration, 400 7th St. SW, Washington, D.C. 20590. Office of Public and Consumer Affairs: (202) 366-9550. For information concerning the National Uniform Crime Reporting Program: Uniform Crime Reports, Criminal Justice Information Services Division, FBI/GRB, Washington, D.C. 20535. Information Dissemination: (202) 324-5015.

Fatal Workplace Injuries Involving Alcohol: 1992

Reported fatalities in the workplace involving alcohol, compared to type of fatal event or exposure and *BAC (blood alcohol concentration) of worker killed. The totals shown here were taken from 1,355 detailed death reports. Those 1,355 reports represented only 25% of all reported job-related deaths in the United States.

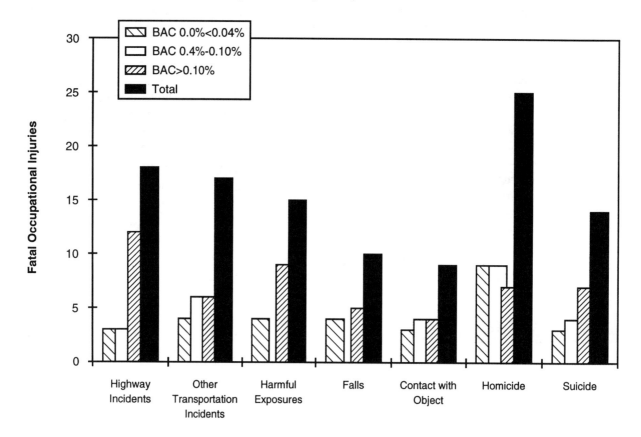

	*BAC 0.01% < 0.04%	*BAC 0.04% – 0.10%	*BAC > 0.10%	TOTAL**
Highway incidents	3	3	12	18
Other transportation incidents	4	6	6	17
Harmful exposures	4	—	9	15
Falls	4	—	5	10
Contact with object	3	4	4	9
Homicide	9	9	7	25
Suicide	3	4	7	14
TOTAL**	32	30	50	108

* BAC is the measure of the amount of alcohol in a person's blood, given in grams per deciliter (g/dL, with 100 grams = one deciliter).
** Numbers do not add because some cases were counted more than once.

Comments These statistics provide insight into the role of alcohol in fatal injuries in the workplace.

In 1992, there were 6,083 job-related deaths in the United States. The Bureau of Labor Statistics' Census of Fatal Occupational Injuries (CFOI) program collected reports from 43 states and the District of Columbia on 5,444 of those deaths. Of the 5,444 reports collected, the CFOI gathered detailed death reports on about one-fourth, or 1,355. Of the 1,355 detailed death reports submitted, 108 (8%) tested positive for alcohol.

The findings from this sample group can be used to make generalizations about the role of alcohol in all job-related deaths in the U.S. Since about 8% of the submitted reports showed alcohol involvement, it can be estimated that throughout the U.S. in 1992 about 500 people were killed on the job due to the effects of alcohol. This generalization assumes that the 1,355 reports for which data was collected are representative of the nation at large.

The blood alcohol concentration (BAC), expressed as a percentage of grams of alcohol per deciliter of blood, serves to indicates how much alcohol is involved in an incident. The National Highway Traffic Safety Administration (NHTSA) considers a traffic fatality to have involved alcohol when the BAC level is at 0.01%. The NHTSA recommends that persons with a BAC of 0.04% be considered alcohol impaired.

The 0.10% level is the legal intoxication level in many states. However, as of 1993, ten states had set the lower level of 0.08% as the legal intoxication threshold.

According to the CFOI report, alcohol, at 68%, was more prevalent in the detailed death reports involving intentional deaths (homicide and suicide), than in unintentional deaths, at 46%. The average BAC, however, was higher in the unintentional deaths (0.113%) than in the intentional ones (0.084%). About 32% of the reports of unintentional deaths involving alcohol had BAC levels of 0.15% or higher.

Source U.S. Department of Labor. Bureau of Labor Statistics. *Census of Fatal Occupational Injuries, 1992.* Washington, D.C.: U.S. Government Printing Office, [1992].

Contact U.S. Department of Labor, Bureau of Labor Statistics, Office of Safety, Health, and Working Conditions, 2 Massachusetts Ave. NE, Washington, D.C. 20212; (202) 606-6175.

Fetal Alcohol Syndrome Rates: 1979–93

Rates per 10,000 births of fetal alcohol syndrome in newborns
due to mother's drinking during pregnancy.

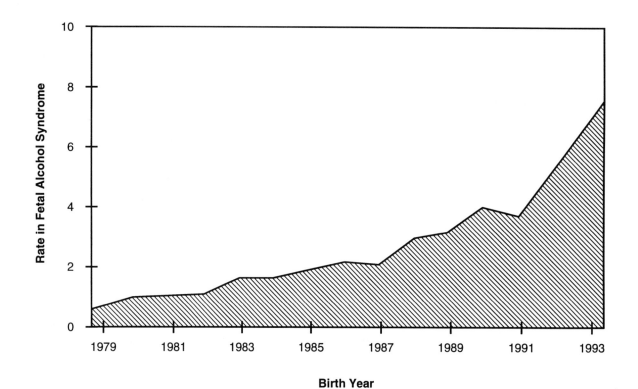

Birth Year

Year	Rate per 10,000 Births
1979	1.0
1980	1.2
1981	1.2
1982	1.2
1983	1.7
1984	1.7
1985	1.9
1986	2.3
1987	2.2
1988	3.0
1989	3.2
1990	4.0
1991	3.7
1992	5.2
1993	6.7

Comments Fetal alcohol syndrome (FAS) is a preventable condition which is characterized by a variety of physical and behavioral traits. These result from the consumption of alcohol by an expectant mother during pregnancy. Some typical features of FAS include diminished growth both before and after birth, telltale abnormal facial features, mental retardation, and central nervous system deficiencies.

According to the national Birth Defects Monitoring Program (BDMP), the rate of reported FAS cases in 1992 was nearly four times that of 1979. In 1993, the BDMP monitored data on approximately 5% of all births (compared with the 30% in 1979); FAS was reported in 126 of 188,905 newborns that year, for a rate of 6.7 per 10,000. During the 1979–93 period, 2,032 FAS cases were reported out of 9,434,560 newborns, giving an overall rate of 2.2 per 10,000 births. The rate for 1993 (6.7 per 10,000 births) was over six times greater than the 1979 rate (1.0 per 10,000 births).

The statistics given here may not give an accurate account of FAS frequency. The increase since 1979 may indicate increased alcohol consumption by pregnant women, or it may be the result of greater awareness and more accurate diagnosis by medical personnel. It is likely that the reported increase is the result of a combination of the two.

Source U.S. Department of Health and Human Services. Public Health Service. Centers for Disease Control and Prevention. "Update: Trends in Fetal alcohol Syndrome– United States," *Morbidity and Mortality Weekly Report* 44, No. 13 (1995): pp. 249–251.

Contact Department of Health and Human Services, Public Health Service, Centers for Disease Control and Prevention, Atlanta, GA 30333. For inquiries about the *Morbidity and Mortality Weekly Report*, call (404) 332-455. The CDC also maintains a World-Wide Web server at http:// www.cdc.gov/.

Alcohol-Induced Deaths: 1979–92

The number of alcohol-induced deaths per year according to gender.

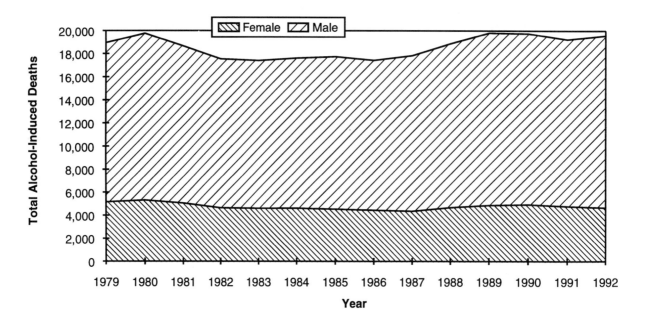

Year	Female	Male
1979	5,163	13,788
1980	5,318	14,447
1981	5,060	13,600
1982	4,638	12,903
1983	4,588	12,812
1984	4,611	12,995
1985	4,525	13,216
1986	4,439	12,986
1987	4,358	13,461
1988	4,666	14,206
1989	4,850	14,960
1990	4,915	14,842
1991	4,766	14,467
1992	4,642	14,926

Comments Every year the Centers for Disease Control and Prevention (CDC) computes mortality (death) statistics for the entire nation. Included are deaths caused directly from drug and alcohol use. These statistics, however, do not include alcohol-related causes like accidents and homicides.

According to the CDC, the causes of death physiologically attributable to alcohol consumption are limited to the following: alcohol psychoses, alcohol dependence syn-drome, nondependent abuse of alcohol, alcoholic polyneuropathy, alcoholic cardiomyopathy, alcoholic gastritis, chronic liver disease and cirrhosis (specified as alcoholic), excessive blood level of alcohol, and accidental poisoning by alcohol.

Many of these causes are related to the voluntary consumption of liquor, but it is not possible to tell how many of the persons who died from alcohol-induced causes were habitual drinkers.

Source Centers for Disease Control and Prevention, "Advance Report of Final Mortal-ity Statistics, 1992," *Monthly Vital Statistics Report,* Vol. 43, No. 6, suppl., [1995], table 21.

Contact U.S. Department of Health and Human Services, Public Health Service, Centers for Disease Control and Prevention, National Center for Health Statistics, 6525 Belcrest Rd., Hyattsville, MD 20782. (301) 436-8500.

dRuGs

Major Federal Drug Control Legislation: 1868–1990

Chronological listing of laws enacted to control illegal drug use in the U.S., classified by the main tactic used.

Year(s)	Major Federal Legislation or International Convention	Regulation & Taxation	Prevention & Education	Prohibition & Criminal Justice	Treatment
1868	Pharmacy Act: required registration of those dispensing drugs	X			
1887–90	Opium importation, domestic cultivation, manufacture, and trafficking limited/prohibited			X	
1906	Pure Food and Drug Act: disallowed adulteration and mislabeling; led to decline of patent medicines	X			
1909	Opium Exclusion Act			X	
1913	International Opium Convention: ratified by U.S. Senate			X	
1914	Harrison Narcotics Act: taxed and regulated sales and distribution of narcotics	X			
1920	Volsted Act: national alcohol prohibition (prohibition ends in 1933)			X	
1922	Narcotic Drugs Import and Export Act: restricted opium imports and exports, expanded role of Customs Department in prohibiting shipments of illegal narcotics into the U.S.			X	
1929	Porter Narcotic Farm Act: established two narcotics hospitals for addicts in federal prisons				X
1937	Marijuana Tax Act	X			
1942	Opium Poppy Control Act			X	
1951	Boggs Act: imposed harsher penalties			X	
1956	Narcotics Control Act: increased penalties and defined sole role of federal government in the suppression of illegal drug activity			X	
1963	Community Mental Health Centers Act: provided first federal assistance to local treatment of addiction under classification of mental illness				X
1965	Drug Abuse Control amendments: regulated depressant and stimulant drugs	X			
1966	Narcotics Addict Rehabilitation Act: fundamental reorientation to the addict				X
1968	Mental Health Centers Act amendments: provided funding specifically for local drug dependence treatment				X
1970	Controlled Substances Act and the Controlled Substances Import and Export Act: created schedules for drugs, altered penalties for violations, and strengthened regulation of the pharmaceutical industry	X		X	
1970	Drug Abuse Education Act		X		
1972	Drug Abuse Office and Treatment Act: established National Institute on Drug Abuse				X
1974	Narcotic Addict Treatment Act: controlled dispensing of methadone				X
1974	Alcohol and Drug Abuse Education Act amendments: targeted prevention and early intervention		X		
1979	Drug Abuse Prevention Treatment and Rehabilitation amendments		X		X
1982	Department of Defense Authorization Act: permits military to operate civilian equipment			X	

[Continued]

Major Federal Drug Control Legislation:1868–1990

[Continued]

Year(s)	Major Federal Legislation or International Convention	Regulation & Taxation	Prevention & Education	Prohibition & Criminal Justice	Treatment
1984	Comprehensive Crime Control Act: amended drug control laws (included civil and criminal forfeiture provisions) and created the National Drug Enforcement Policy Board			X	
1986	Anti-Drug Abuse Act: contained enforcement provisions, state assistance, and research provisions; also established White House Conference for a Drug-Free America and created Office for Substance Abuse Prevention (OSAP)		X	X	
1988	Anti-Drug Abuse Act: created Office of National Drug Abuse Policy and focused on penalties for trafficking, on new offenses and regulations, and on reducing foreign production and trafficking; OSAP expands to education and early intervention		X	X	
1990	Crime Control Act: contained 37 titles including drug-free school zones, rural drug enforcement, drug grants, and regulation of precursor chemicals	X		X	
TOTAL		7	5	14	7

Comments Since the 1860s, governments at the state and federal level have used a variety of policies and tactics to address a changing drug problem. Major federal drug control efforts are listed here. The classification of these policies by tactics is somewhat subjective. It is designed to provide an overview to the history of drug control efforts in the U.S.

A policy of *regulation* establishes control over the distribution, possession, and use of certain substances, and specifies the circumstances under which substances can be legally distributed and used. Similarly, the tactic of *taxation* requires those who produce, distribute, or possess drugs to pay a fee based on the volume or value of the drugs.

Prevention activities are educational efforts to inform potential drug users about the health, legal, and other risks of using drugs. *Criminal justice* activities include enforcement, prosecution, and sentencing activities to apprehend, convict, and punish drug offenders. *Treatment* focuses on individuals whose drug use has caused them medical, psychological, economic, and social problems.

Source U. S. Department of Justice. Office of Justice Programs. Bureau of Justice Statistics. *Drugs, Crime, and the Justice System, a National Report from the Bureau of Justice Statistics, December 1992, NCJ-133652.* Washington, D.C.: U.S. Government Printing Office, [1992], pp.78–83.

Contact Bureau of Justice Statistics Clearinghouse, Box 6000, Rockville, MD 20850; (800) 732-3277. Drugs & Crime Data Center & Clearinghouse, 1600 Research Blvd., Rockville, MD 20850; (800) 666-3332.

World Production of Three Illegal Drug Crops: 1987–91

World production (in metric tons) of three major agricultural crops used to produce illegal drugs.

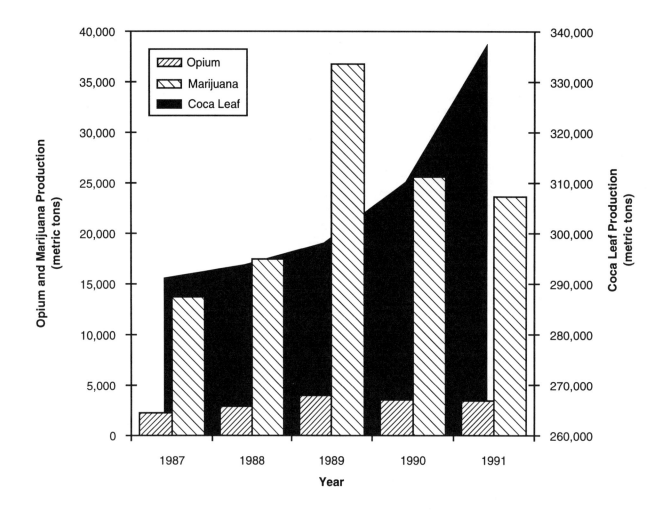

	1987	1988	1989	1990	1991*
Opium	2,242	2,881	3,948	3,520	3,429
Marijuana	13,693	17,455	36,755	25,600	23,650
Coca leaf	291,100	293,700	298,070	310,170	337,100

* Estimated.

Comments This graph shows the estimated world production of three types of agricultural crops used to produce illegal drugs: opium (used to make heroin), marijuana, and coca leaf (used for cocaine). Southeast Asia, including Burma (also known as Myanmar), Laos, and Thailand, accounts for about three-fourths of the estimated world opium supply. Most of the remainder coming from Afghanistan, Iran, and Pakistan.

Most marijuana consumed in the U.S. comes either from other sources in the Western Hemisphere (Colombia, Mexico, Jamaica, Belize, Puerto Rico) or from "homegrown" activities in the U.S. itself. Climate and soil conditions are the primary determinants for the agricultural production of these crops, but social and political factors are important as well.

The illegal drug crops are usually grown on small independent farms. Such crops may be the only dependable source of farm income. These local growers, however, rarely become wealthy. Many are members of social or ethnic groups that are outside the official power structure, such as the Kurds in the Middle East and the Hmong in Southeast Asia. In some areas, coca leaf and opium poppies have traditionally been grown and used for medicinal purposes or as part of the local culture. In Burma and Peru, for example, this type of cultivation and use has existed for centuries.

Since these growers often operate outside the legal economy, it is not possible to know exactly how much of these crops are actually produced. It is possible, however, to gather enough information to make an estimate. This graph follows the trends in those estimates from 1987 to 1991.

According to the graph, the yearly production amounts for opium and marijuana (measured by the scale on the left) are much less than the production of coca leaf (as measured by the scale on the right). Two different scales for metric tons are used in order to simultaneously compare the trends for the three drug crops while accommodating for the large gap. For the years shown in the chart, estimated coca leaf production has risen swiftly since 1987, while opium and marijuana production peaked in 1989.

The reason for the high tonnage of coca leaf production is that extensive processing and refining is required to make cocaine. The coca leaves are first converted into a coca base, then to a cocaine base, and then finally to powdered cocaine. Opium requires less refining (and marijuana little to none) and therefore needs less of the raw product to produce the drug for consumption. Since cocaine production requires so much refining with waste generated at each stage, it is more efficient for cocaine producers to refine the drug close to where the coca leaves are grown, rather than transport the heavy coca leaves.

Source U. S. Department of Justice. Office of Justice Programs. Bureau of Justice Statistics. *Drugs, Crime, and the Justice System, a National Report from the Bureau of Justice Statistics, December 1992, NCJ-133652.* Washington, D.C.: U.S. Government Printing Office, [1992], p. 36. Primary source: U.S. Department of State, Bureau of International Narcotics Matters, *International Narcotics Control Strategy Report,* March 1991, p. 22.

Contact Bureau of Justice Statistics Clearinghouse, Box 6000, Rockville, MD 20850; (800) 732-3277. Drugs & Crime Data Center & Clearinghouse, 1600 Research Blvd., Rockville, MD 20850; (800) 666-3332.

Worldwide Production of Cocaine: 1992 and 1993

The estimated potential net production of cocaine, given by cultivation (number of hectares devoted to growing coca plants) and production (quantity of harvested coca leaf).

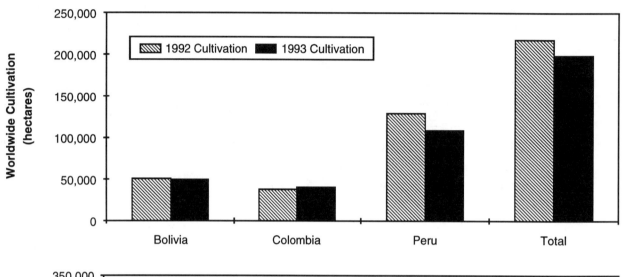

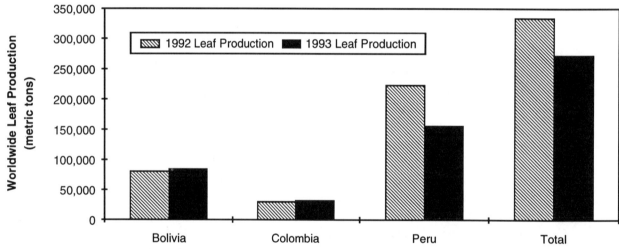

Country	1992 Cultivation (hectares)	1993 Cultivation (hectares)	1992 Leaf Production (metric tons)	1993 Leaf Production (metric tons)
Bolivia	50,649	49,600	80,300	84,400
Colombia	38,059	40,493	29,600	31,700
Peru	129,100	108,800	223,000	155,500
Ecuador	—	—	100	100
TOTAL	217,808	198,893	333,900	271,700

Comments The cocaine consumed in the U.S. is grown in several South American countries. These histograms (bar graphs) illustrate the total cultivation and leaf production amounts for 1992 and 1993. The cultivation statistics refer to the area of land (1 hectare = 2.471 acres) devoted to the production of coca plants. The production statistics describe the quantity of harvested coca leaf. Leaf production for Ecuador is not included in the graphs because of its low amount relative to the other countries.

According to the graphs, both the total area cultivated and the total leaf production amounts fell in 1993 from 1992. Since fewer hectares were cultivated in 1993 than in 1992, it would imply that the leaf production in 1993 was less than in 1992. The decline in the cultivated area, however, may or may not be the only reason why production dropped. Based on the information presented here, it is not possible to know exactly why the total leaf production declined. The drop in cultivation is probably part of the reason, however. According to the DEA, the cultivation dropped in 1993 principally because some fields in Peru were abandoned. These Peruvian coca fields had become infested with a naturally occurring fungus which made it impossible to grow coca plants. Soil depletion and the movement of farmers to safer areas also contributed to the drop in cultivation.

Not all of the production is sent to the U.S. market; some is consumed within the producing country and some is destined for the European market. In 1993, the Office on National Drug Control Policy estimated that 243–340 metric tons of cocaine was available to the U.S. market, down from 376–539 metric tons in 1992.

Source Office of National Drug Control Policy. Executive Office of the President of the United States. *National Drug Control Strategy, Strengthening Communities' Response to Drugs and Crime, February 1995.* Washington, D.C.: U.S. Government Printing Office, [1995], p. 45. Primary source: U.S. Department of State, *International Narcotics Control Strategy Report,* 1994.

Contact Department of State, Bureau of International Narcotics Matters, 2201 C St. NW, Washington, D.C. 20520. Public Affairs: (202) 647-6575. Executive Office of the President of the United States, Office of National Drug Control Policy, Washington, D.C. 20500; (202) 395-6700. Drugs & Crime Data Center & Clearinghouse, 1600 Research Blvd., Rockville, MD 20850; (800)666-3332.

Worldwide Production of Opium: 1988–93

The potential net production of opium (in metric tons) derived
from opium poppies, by nations where they are grown.

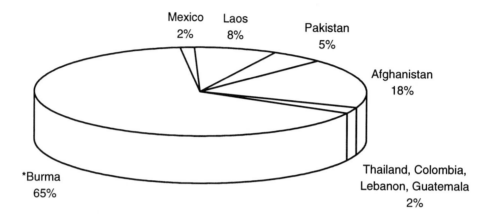

Mexico 2%   Laos 8%   Pakistan 5%

Afghanistan 18%

Thailand, Colombia, Lebanon, Guatemala 2%

*Burma 65%

	1988	1989	1990	1991	1992	1993
Afghanistan	750	585	415	570	640	685
Pakistan	205	130	165	180	175	140
Total, Southwest Asia	955	715	580	750	815	825
Burma	1,280	2,430	2,255	2,350	2,280	2,575
Laos	255	380	275	265	230	180
Thailand	25	50	40	35	24	42
Total, Southeast Asia	1,560	2,860	2,570	2,650	2,534	2,797
Colombia	—	—	—	27	20	20
Lebanon	NA	45	32	34	—	4
Guatemala	8	12	13	17	—	4
Mexico	67	66	62	41	40	49
Total, Americas and Lebanon	75	123	107	119	60	77
TOTAL	2,590	3,698	3,257	3,519	3,409	3,699

* Also known as Myanmar.

Comments The table and pie chart shown here indicate which areas of the world and which specific nations produce opium poppies. Opium poppies are consumed in the form of opium, morphine, and heroin all over the world. According to the table, the world's opium supply rose during 1988 to 1993 and came primarily from Southeast Asia.

Upon closer analysis of each individual nation shown in the pie chart, it becomes obvious that Burma (also known as Myanmar) most recently accounted for the greatest portion of the world's opium supply. The market for heroin in the U.S. is mainly supplied by Southeast Asia. According to the DEA's Heroin Signature Report Program in 1992, Southeast Asia was determined to be the origin of 68% of all heroin analyzed; South America,

15%; Southwest Asia, 9%; and Mexico, 8%. Information on illegal production in some countries is sometimes unclear, especially since opium poppy fields are often in remote areas far from governmental control. Opium can be grown to supply legitimate pharmaceutical needs. For example, poppies are legally grown and cultivated in Turkey under strict government controls.

In Afghanistan, the DEA believed that actual opium production may have exceeded 900 metric tons during 1992 and 1993, but was not able to corroborate this belief. Moreover, the U.S. government believes that some 35–75 metric tons of opium gum is produced annually in Iran, although there is no solid information regarding Iranian opium production.

Source Office of National Drug Control Policy. Executive Office of the President of the United States. *National Drug Control Strategy, Strengthening Communities' Response to Drugs and Crime, February* *1995.* Washington, D.C.: U.S. Government Printing Office, [1995], p. 47. Primary source: U.S. Department of State, *International Narcotics Control Strategy Report,* 1994.

Contact Department of State, Bureau of International Narcotics Matters, 2201 C St. NW, Washington, D.C. 20520. Public Affairs: (202) 647-6575. Executive Office of the President of the United States, Office of National Drug Control Policy, Washington, D.C. 20500;(202) 395-6700. Drugs & Crime Data Center & Clearinghouse, 1600 Research Blvd., Rockville, MD 20850; (800)666-3332.

Worldwide Production of Marijuana: 1988–93

The potential net production of marijuana (in metric tons),
given by nations where the plants are grown (excluding the U.S.).

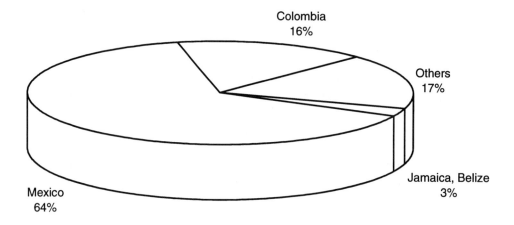

	1988	1989	1990	1991	1992	1993
Mexico	5,655	30,200	19,715	7,775	7,795	6,280
Colombia	7,775	2,800	1,500	1,500	1,500	4,125
Jamaica	405	190	825	641	263	502
Belize	120	65	60	49	0	0
Others	3,500	3,500	3,500	3,500	3,500	3,500
TOTAL	17,455	36,755	25,600	13,465	13,058	14,407

Comments

This chart shows the potential net production of marijuana by four countries in the Americas. The information shown here excludes potential net production by the U.S., where marijuana is produced in remote small outdoor plots and improvised greenhouses. Other countries where some marijuana is produced include Angola, Cambodia, Canada, India, Laos, Nepal, Pakistan, Panama, Russia, Thailand, and Vietnam. According to these statistics, the total potential net production in the Americas has risen or fallen mainly due to Mexico's role. Colombia has played a secondary, but important part.

Source

Office of National Drug Control Policy. Executive Office of the President of the United States. *National Drug Control Strategy, Strengthening Communities' Response to Drugs and Crime, February 1995.* Washington, D.C.: U.S. Government Printing Office, [1995], p. 147. Primary source: U.S. Department of State, *International Narcotics Control Strategy Report, 1994.*

Contact

Department of State, Bureau of International Narcotics Matters, 2201 C St. NW, Washington, D.C. 20520. Public Affairs: (202) 647-6575. Executive Office of the President of the United States, Office of National Drug Control Policy, Washington, D.C. 20500; (202) 395-6700. Drugs & Crime Data Center & Clearinghouse, 1600 Research Blvd., Rockville, MD; 20850; (800)666-3332.

Worldwide Production of Hashish: 1988–93

The potential net production of hashish, a drug made from the cannabis plant,
given by production in several nations.

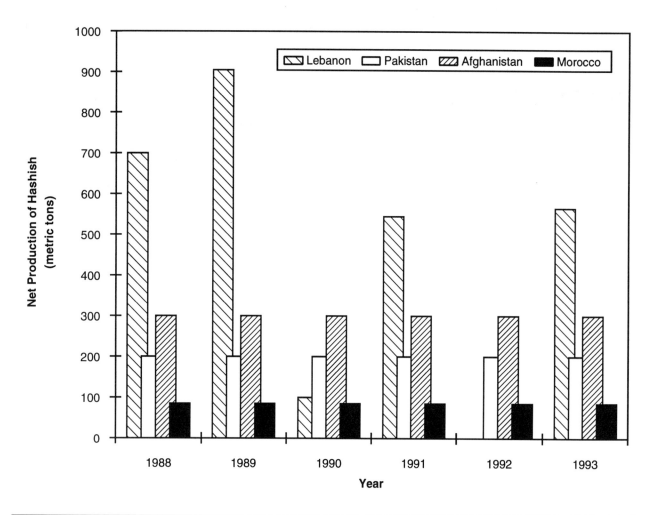

	1988	1989	1990	1991	1992	1993
Lebanon	700	905	100	545	—	565
Pakistan	200	200	200	200	200	200
Afghanistan	300	300	300	300	300	300
Morocco	85	85	85	85	85	85
TOTAL	1,285	1,490	685	1,130	585	1,150

Comments Most of the world's hashish production (a drug, like marijuana, made from the cannabis plant) originates in the Middle East. Hashish oil is produced through a repeated cycle of extracting the THC-rich resin from the flowering tops of the female cannabis plant and discarding the fibrous plant material. Hashish typically is smoked, chewed, or drunk for its mind-altering effects. Significant amounts of hashish are neither produced nor consumed in the U.S. Of the four hashish-producing nations listed here, only one (Lebanon) had varying production levels of hashish during the 1988–93 period. Annual production amounts for Afghanistan, Pakistan, and Morocco remained constant.

Source Office of National Drug Control Policy. Executive Office of the President of the United States. *National Drug Control Strategy, Strengthening Communities' Response to Drugs and Crime, February 1995.* Washington, D.C.: U.S. Government Printing Office, [1995], p. 147. Primary source: U.S. Department of State, *International Narcotics Control Strategy Report, 1994.*

Contact Department of State, Bureau of International Narcotics Matters, 2201 C St. NW, Washington, D.C. 20520. Public Affairs: (202) 647-6575. Executive Office of the President of the United States, Office of National Drug Control Policy, Washington, D.C. 20500; (202) 395-6700. Drugs & Crime Data Center & Clearinghouse, 1600 Research Blvd., Rockville, MD 20850; (800)666-3332.

Drugs Smuggled into the U.S.: 1986

The proportion of illegal drugs smuggled into the U.S., given by method of transportation from country of origin.

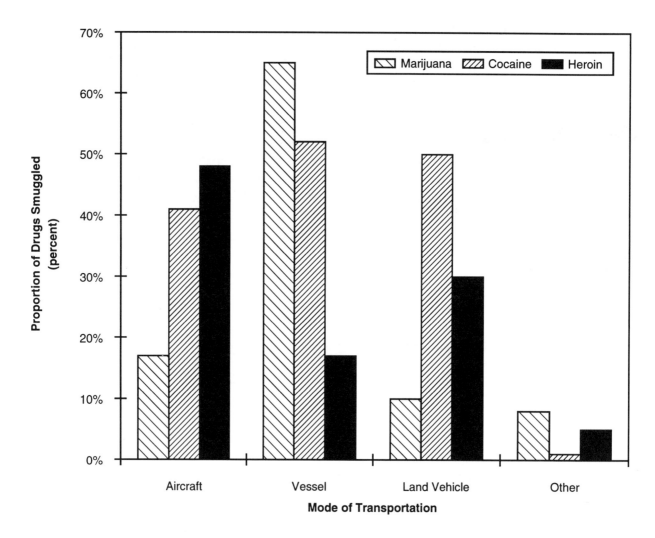

Mode of Transport	Marijuana	Cocaine	Heroin
Aircraft	17%	41%	48%
Vessel	65%	52%	17%
Land vehicle	10%	5%	30%
Other	8%	1%	5%
TOTAL	100%	100%*	100%

* Does not add due to rounding.

Comments The flow of illegal drugs into the U.S. is accomplished by various forms of smuggling. The U.S. has 88,633 miles of coastline, 7,500 miles of borders with Canada and Mexico, and 300 ports of entry. It is very difficult to stop illegal drugs from coming into the country. In 1990/91, for example, more than 438 million people, 128 million vehicles, 157,000 vessels, 586,000 aircraft, and 3.5 million containers entered the U.S.

This chart shows how the method of drug smuggling varied by drug in 1986. The term "aircraft" refers to all public and private airplanes and helicopters; "vessel" includes private and commercial boats and ships; "land vehicle" refers to passenger and commercial cars, trucks, and motorcycles; and "other" refers to drugs smuggled personally by an individual, by animal, or by any other method.

According to the chart, about two-thirds of all marijuana was smuggled into the U.S. by boat, with land vehicles and aircraft used much less frequently. For heroin, however, aircraft was used for about half of the smuggling, while most of the remaining heroin was smuggled across the border by car or truck.

The preferred methods for smuggling cocaine are almost exclusively by vessel or aircraft; all other methods accounted for less than 10%.

The method of transportation depends largely on where the drug is produced. For example, much of the marijuana brought into the U.S. comes from Central and South America. Since marijuana is inherently a bulky agricultural substance, it is cost effective for drug traffickers to rely on vessels for smuggling. Since cocaine comes primarily from South America, aircraft are used more extensively. When weight is a transportation concern, air transport is generally more expensive than of land or water. Since cocaine is less bulky and each kilogram can generate more profit than a kilogram of marijuana or heroin, the added cost of air transport can be absorbed by the greater profits associated with cocaine trafficking.

Unlike marijuana and cocaine, land vehicle smuggling accounts for a significant proportion of the heroin brought into the U.S. Heroin coming overseas from Asia and the Middle East is transported by air and water.

Source U.S. Department of Justice. Office of Justice Programs. Bureau of Justice Statistics. *Drugs, Crime, and the Justice System, A National Report from the Bureau of Justice Statistics, December 1992, NCJ-* *133652.* Washington, D.C.: U.S. Government Printing Office, [1992], p. 44. Primary source: General Accounting Office, *Drug Smuggling: Large Amounts of Illegal Drugs not Seized by Federal Authorities*, June 1987, p. 16.

Contact General Accounting Office, National Security and International Affairs Division, 441 G St. NW, Washington, D.C. 20548. Public Affairs: (202) 275-2812.

Individuals Reporting Illegal Drug Use: 1993

Percentages of persons in households who reported using specific illegal drugs
in the past month, past year, and lifetime.

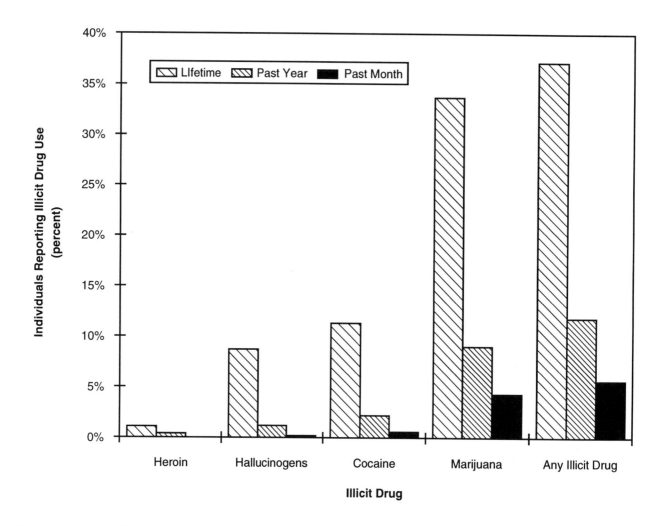

	Heroin	Hallucinogens	Cocaine	Marijuana	Any Illicit Drug
Past month	0.0%	0.2%	0.6%	4.3%	5.6%
Past year	0.1%	1.2%	2.2%	9.0%	11.8%
Lifetime	1.1%	8.7%	11.3%	33.7%	37.2%

Comments   As of 1993, some 37.2% of the civilian noninstitutionalized population of the U.S. (aged 12 and older) reported illicit drug use in their lifetimes. According to the 1993 National Household Survey on Drug Abuse (NHSDA), more than 77 million people reported that they had used illicit drugs at some time during their lives. Of those, 70 million people reported using marijuana, 23 million had used cocaine, 18 million had used hallucinogens, 4 million had tried crack cocaine, and more than 2 million had tried heroin.

This bar chart gives some perspective as to the number of illicit drug users. For instance, by looking at the category "any illicit drug," one can surmise that of all the people who ever used an illicit drug, fewer than one-third of them had done so within the past year. Of those who had taken illicit drugs within the past year, just under half of them had done so within the past month. The 5.6% of "past month users is included in the 11.8% of past year" users, which is a portion of the 37.2% of "lifetime" users. Marijuana was the most frequently used illicit drug, with 33.7% of the civilian noninstitutionalized population reporting its use some time during their lives. Marijuana often is the first illegal drug used by an individual; it commonly serves as a bridge in the transition from using legal substances like tobacco and alcohol, to the use of more potent illegal drugs like cocaine and heroin.

It is important to remember that the validity of this survey, like any other, relies on the honesty of the respondents. It is therefore likely that the actual use of these drugs by the total U.S. population is higher, both because survey respondents underreport drug use and because chronic, hardcore drug users probably are not well represented in drug prevalence surveys.

Source   Office of National Drug Control Policy. Executive Office of the President of the United States. *National Drug Control Strategy, Strengthening Communities' Response to Drugs and Crime, February 1995.* Washington, D.C.: U.S. Government Printing Office, [1995], p. 18. Primary source: Substance Abuse and Mental Health Services Administration, *National Household Survey on Drug Abuse,* 1993.

Contact   U.S. Department of Health and Human Services, Public Health Service, Substance Abuse and Mental Health Services Administration, 5600 Fishers Lane, Rockville, MD 20857; (301) 443-3875.

Cocaine Use and Overall Illegal Drug Use: 1979–93

Trends in frequency of cocaine use or use of any illegal drug, by numbers (in millions) of persons.

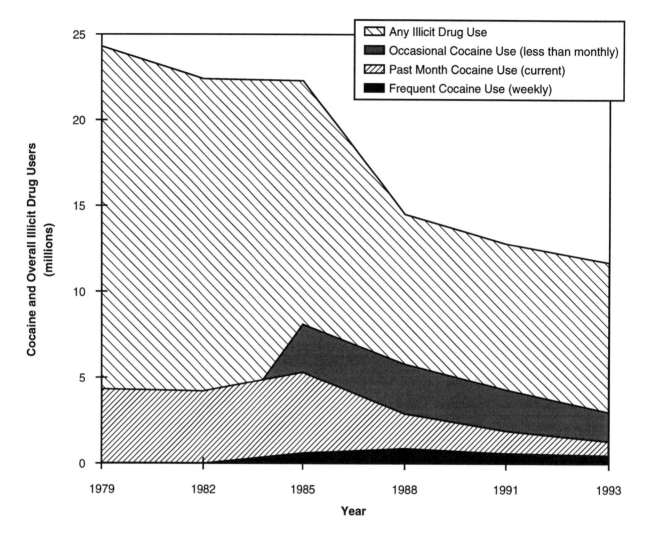

	1979	1982	1985	1988	1991	1993
Frequent (weekly) cocaine use	—	—	0.6	0.9	0.6	0.5
Past month (current) cocaine use	4.3	4.2	5.3	2.9	1.9	1.3
Occasional (less than monthly) cocaine use	—	—	8.1	5.8	4.3	3.0
Any illicit drug use	24.3	22.4	22.3	14.5	12.8	11.7

Comments This chart shows the trends in illicit drug use, as estimated by household surveys. The categories for frequent and occasional cocaine use in 1979 and 1982 are blank because no data for those questions were gathered in those years. Consequently, it is not possible to know exactly what the trends were in those years. The category "any illicit drug use" refers to lifetime use of any illegal drugs, and is the most inclusive of the four categories shown.

According to the chart, from 1979 to 1993, the number of individuals who ever used illicit drugs—even once—fell by over 50%, from 24.3 million to 11.7 million. Although the number of individuals who ever used illegal drugs fell somewhat from 1979 to 1985, the number of current cocaine users rose and peaked in 1985. From 1985 to 1993, the number of current cocaine users fell by about 75% from 5.3 million to 1.3 million. The number of hardcore (weekly) cocaine users is small compared to current and occasional cocaine users. However, the number of individuals who were frequent cocaine users has been fairly consistent, despite a decline from 0.9 million in 1988 to 0.5 million in 1993.

Source Office of National Drug Control Policy. Executive Office of the President of the United States. *National Drug Control Strategy, Strengthening Communities' Response to Drugs and Crime, February 1995.* Washington, D.C.: U.S. Government Printing Office, [1995], table B-3, p. 139. Primary source: National Institute on Drug Abuse (1979–91), and Substance Abuse and Mental Health Services Administration, (1992–93), *National Household Survey on Drug Abuse,* 1993.

Contact U.S. Department of Health and Human Services, Public Health Service, Substance Abuse and Mental Health Services Administration, National Institute on Drug Abuse, 5600 Fishers Lane, Rockville, MD 20857; (301) 443-6487. Public Relations: (301) 443-1124. National Clearinghouse for Alcohol and Drug Information: (800) 729-6686.

Estimated Cocaine and Heroin Users: 1988–93

Approximate number of cocaine and heroin users and proportions of casual (less than once a week) and heavy (at least once a week) users.

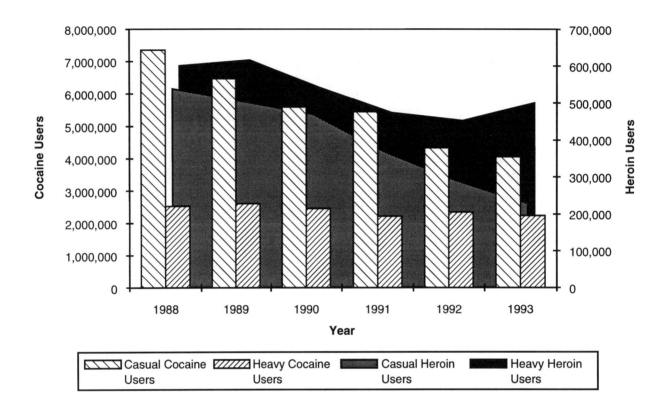

Cocaine User Populations						
	1988	1989	1990	1991	1992	1993
Casual users	7,347,000	6,466,000	5,585,000	5,440,000	4,331,000	4,054,000
Heavy users	2,526,000	2,611,000	2,456,000	2,219,000	2,349,000	2,238,000
Heroin User Populations						
Casual users	539,000	504,000	470,000	368,000	290,000	229,000
Heavy users	601,000	616,000	542,000	474,000	452,000	500,000

Comments These tables and chart present estimates of the numbers of Americans who use cocaine and heroin, and what proportions are casual and heavy users. *Casual users* are defined as individuals that use the drug less than once per week, while *heavy users* are defined as those who use the drug at least once per week.

For cocaine, the total number of users has fallen since the late 1980s, due to a nearly 45% drop in the number of casual users; the number of heavy users has remained fairly consistent, only dropping by just under 12% during the six-year cycle. The number of casual users of heroin fell by nearly 60% from 1988 to 1993, while the number of heavy users dropped by less than 20% during that same period. These statistics imply that casual use fluctuates from one year to the next more than heavy drug use.

Individuals who become heavy drug users may be less willing or able to give up their habits. Another reason that might explain the consistency of the populations of heavy cocaine and heroin users is the notion that casual users will become heavy users rather than heavy users reverting to casual use.

By this explanation, the category "heavy users" becomes the final category of analysis. If an individual uses cocaine or heroin more than once per week, regardless of increasing frequency of use, there is no way to categorize any further severity of drug use by that person. In other words, if the category "heavy users" were subdivided (e.g., "moderately heavy," "very heavy," "extremely heavy") it could give a more detailed view of the numbers of individuals using cocaine and heroin.

Source Office of National Drug Control Policy. Executive Office of the President of the United States. *National Drug Control Strategy, Strengthening Communities' Response to Drugs and Crime, February* *1995.* Washington, D.C.: U.S. Government Printing Office, [1995], table B-4, p. 139. Primary source: Abt Associates, Inc., *What America's Users Spend on Illegal Drugs*, 1988–93, in press.

Contact Executive Office of the President of the United States, Office of National Drug Control Policy, Washington, D.C. 20500; (202) 395-6700.

Annual Cocaine Consumption: 1972–92

Trends in cocaine use by hardcore (heavy) and casual (light) users in the U.S.

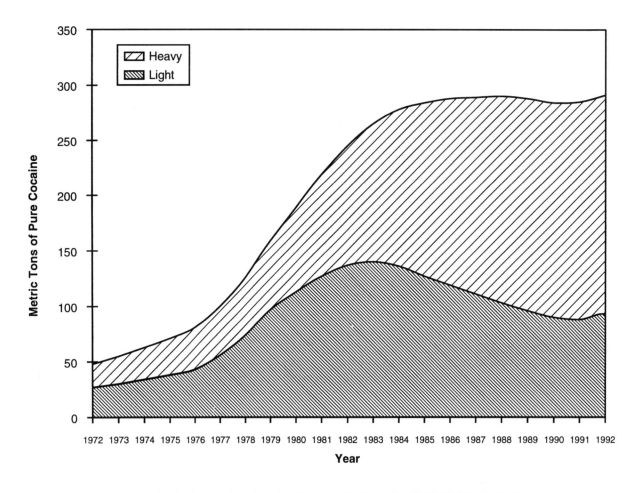

Year	Consumption (metric tons)		Year	Consumption (metric tons)	
	Light	Heavy		Light	Heavy
1972	27	21	1983	140	125
1973	30	25	1984	136	142
1974	34	29	1985	127	157
1975	38	33	1986	119	169
1976	43	38	1987	111	178
1977	56	44	1988	103	187
1978	74	52	1989	96	192
1979	97	62	1990	90	194
1980	113	76	1991	88	197
1981	127	92	1992	90	201
1982	137	108			

Comments Chronic or hardcore users currently account for the majority of cocaine consumption in the U.S. The Office of National Drug Control Policy has estimated that the number of hardcore drug users has remained relatively unchanged since 1988. The Office also estimated the total population of chronic, hardcore drug users in 1993 to be 2.7 million, with about 2.1 million people using primarily cocaine and 600,000 using mostly heroin. The chronic users represent about 20% of the drug-using population but consume about two-thirds of the total cocaine in the U.S.

In the early 1970s, the ratio of hardcore hardcore users to casual users was about the same. However, during the 1970s, casual use of cocaine grew much faster than hardcore use. In the early 1980s, however, this trend reversed with consumption by casual users peaking in 1983, while hardcore cocaine use steadily rose. When casual consumption peaked in 1983, the ratio of consumption by hardcore and casual users was again about the same, comparable to the early 1970s. However, after 1983, hardcore use rose slightly and hit a plateau of about 280 million metric tons throughout the rest of the 1980s. Casual consumption continued falling, dropping to less than 100 metric tons per year by the late 1980s.

Source Office of National Drug Control Policy. Executive Office of the President of the United States. *National Drug Control Strategy, Strengthening Communities' Response to Drugs and Crime, February 1995.* Washington, D.C.: U.S. Government Printing Office, [1995], pp.17–21. Primary source: RAND Corporation, *Modeling the Demand for Cocaine,* 1994.

Contact RAND Corporation, Domestic Research Division, 1700 Main St. P.O. Box 2138, Santa Monica, CA, 90406; (213) 393-0411. Executive Office of the President of the United States, Office of National Drug Control Policy, Washington, D.C. 20500; (202) 395-6700.

Drug Use Among High School Seniors: 1991–94

Trends in drug use by high school seniors over a 4-year period,
listed by percentage who reported ever using a specific drug.

	Class of 1991	Class of 1992	Class of 1993	Class of 1994
Any illicit drug	44.1	40.7	42.9	45.6
Marijuana/hashish	36.7	32.6	35.3	38.2
Inhalants	17.6	16.6	17.4	17.7
Inhalants adjusted	18.0	17.0	17.7	18.3
Amyl and butyl nitrates	1.6	1.5	1.4	1.7
Hallucinogens	9.6	9.2	10.9	11.4
Hallucinogens adjusted	10.0	9.4	11.3	11.7
LSD	8.8	8.6	10.3	10.5
PCP	2.9	2.4	2.9	2.8
Cocaine	7.8	6.1	6.1	5.9
Crack	3.1	2.6	2.6	3.0
Other cocaine	7.0	5.3	5.4	5.2
Heroin	0.9	1.2	1.1	1.2
Other opiates	6.6	6.1	6.4	6.6
Stimulants*	15.4	13.9	15.1	15.7
Crystal methamphetamine	3.4	2.9	3.1	3.4
Sedatives*	6.7	6.1	6.4	7.3
Barbiturates*	6.2	5.5	6.3	7.0
Methaqualone*	1.3	1.6	0.8	1.4
Tranquilizers*	7.2	6.0	6.4	6.6

* Only use not under a doctor's order included.

Comments These statistics come from a yearly survey taken which asks students about their frequency of drug and alcohol use. By polling a group of students and making observations based on their responses, it is possible to adapt these observations to fit the entire student population. For example, in 1991, there were 15,483 high school seniors surveyed out of over 2.5 million seniors in the U.S. Although the sample size represents less than 1% of the total population of high school seniors, it is still possible to make observations based on the sample. This method of gathering information based on sampling is commonly used in many everyday aspects of decision-making by those in government, medicine, insurance, and marketing. Each profession that uses this method, however, focuses on its own unique problems and priorities.

In this example, the drug use of four consecutive classes of high school seniors shows that during 1991 to 1994, drug use among 12th graders rose steadily. By limiting the data to these four years however, the reader is not made aware of the fact that drug use by high school seniors has been falling gradually over the long run from its peak of 65.6% in 1979. The 40.7% of 1992 is the lowest value of all during 1975–1994. Seventeen different drugs are shown. The highest responses in the period from 1991 to 1994 are for marijuana, stimulants, inhalants, and hallucinogens.

The categories "inhalants adjusted" and "hallucinogens adjusted" refer to a change of reporting where it was believed the form of the questionnaire impeded accuracy. Inhalants were adjusted for underreporting amyl and butyl nitrates, and hallucinogens were adjusted for underreporting PCP. Some opiates, stimulants, barbiturates, methaqualone, and tranquilizers are legal but controlled substances. The use of these drugs by seniors under a physician's order for legitimate medical purposes was not included.

Source U.S. Department of Health and Human Services. Public Health Service. Substance Abuse and Mental Health Services Administration. National Institute on Drug Abuse. *Monitoring the Future Study, 1975–1994: National High School Senior Drug Abuse Survey,* 1994, p. 2.

Contact U.S. Department of Health and Human Services, Public Health Service, Substance Abuse and Mental Health Services Administration, National Institute on Drug Abuse, 5600 Fishers Lane, Rockville, MD 20857; (301) 443-6487. Public Relations: (301) 443-1124. National Clearinghouse for Alcohol and Drug Information: (800) 729-6686.

Effects of Illegal Drugs

Drug Type	Short-term Effects		Duration of Acute Effects	DEA View of Risk of Dependence
	Desired	Other		
Heroin	Euphoria Pain reduction	Respiratory depression Nausea Drowsiness	3 to 6 hours	Physical -high Psychological -high
Cocaine	Excitement Euphoria Increased alertness, wakefulness	Increased blood pressure Increased respiratory rate Nausea Cold sweats Twitching Headache	1 to 2 hours	Physical -possible Psychological -high
Crack Cocaine	Same as cocaine More rapid high than cocaine	Same as cocaine	About 5 minutes	Same as cocaine
Marijuana	Euphoria Relaxation	Accelerated heartbeat Impairment of perception, judgment, fine motor skills, and memory	2 to 4 hours	Physical -unknown Psychological -moderate
Amphetamines	Euphoria Excitement Increased alertness, wakeful-ness	Increased blood pressure Increased pulse rate Misnaming Loss of appetite	2 to 4 hours	Physical -possible Psychological -high
LSD	Illusions and hallucinations Excitement Euphoria	Poor perception of time and distance Acute anxiety, restless-ness, sleeplessness Sometimes depression	8 to 12 hours	Physical -none Psychological -unknown

Comments People use illicit drugs to induce a variety of effects: mood change, excitement, relaxation, pleasure, numbness, stimulation, or sedation. This table shows how different drugs compare in terms of what effects they produce, how long the effects last, and the Drug Enforcement Agency's assessment on the potential for physical and psychological dependence for each drug.

Some drugs are taken in the belief that they will enhance physical or mental performance or give the user spiritual enlightenment. Most illicit drugs are taken purely for their mind-altering effects. Some drugs, like heroin, have very limited legitimate medical uses. Other drugs—like stimulants, sedatives, tranquilizers, and analgesics—have defined, specific medical uses including sedation, weight control, and pain control. These drugs are controlled substances available only by prescription. Because these prescription-type psychotherapeutic drugs can produce potent mind-altering effects, they are used by substanse abusers. Consequently, they can become a valuable commodity for those wishing to distribute or consume such a drug illegally.

Many commonly abused drugs are sought for the euphoria they produce, but they are also used to produce other types of mind-altering effects. Examples of drug use for other desired effects include: heroin, to reduce pain; cocaine, to produce excitement; marijuana, to promote feelings of relaxation and intoxication; and stimulants, to increase alertness.

Drug use may also be a symptom of (or response to) a psychiatric disorder. It is common for many people with substance abuse problems to have affective, anxiety, or personality disorders; the converse is true as well. Some people believe that drug users are actually attempting self-medication (either knowingly or subconciously) for their psychiatric disorders. For example, a person who is depressed may use drugs to elevate his or her mood; a person suffering from severe anxiety may seek relief by the fear-reducing and relaxing effects of some drugs.

Source U.S. Department of Justice. Office of Justice Programs. Bureau of Justice Statistics. *Drugs, Crime, and the Justice System, A National Report from the Bureau of Justice Statistics, December 1992, NCJ-133652.* Washington, D.C.: U.S. Government Printing Office, [1992], p. 20. Primary source: National Institute on Drug Abuse, "Heroin," *NIDA Capsules,* August 1986; Drug Enforcement Administration, *Drugs of Abuse,* 1989; G.R. Gay, "Clinical Management of Acute and Chronic Cocaine Poisoning: Concepts, Components, and Configuration," *Annals of Emergency Medicine,* (1982) 11, no. 10: pp. 562–572 as cited in NIDA, Dale D. Chitwood, "Patterns and Consequences of Cocaine Use," in *Cocaine Use in America: Epidemiologic and Clinical Perspectives,* Nicholas J. Kozel and Edgar H. Adams, eds., NIDA Research Monograph 61, 1985; NIDA, James A. Inciardi, "Crack-Cocaine in Miami," in *The Epidemiology of Cocaine Use and Abuse,* Susan Schober and Charles Schade, eds., NIDA Research Monograph 110, 1991; and NIDA, "Marijuana," *NIDA Capsules,* August 1986.

Contact U.S. Department of Health and Human Services, Public Health Service, Substance Abuse and Mental Health Services Administration, National Institute on Drug Abuse, 5600 Fishers Lane, Rockville, MD 20857; (301) 443-6487. Public Relations: (301) 443-1124. National Clearinghouse for Alcohol and Drug Information: (800) 729-6686. Drug Enforcement Administration, 600-700 Army Navy Dr., Arlington, VA 22202. Public Affairs: (202) 307-7977.

Drug Ranking Schedule of the DEA

Rankings of specific drugs by the Drug Enforcement Administration (DEA)
according to potency, usefulness, and potential for abuse.

DEA Schedule	Examples of Drugs Covered	Some of the Effects	Medical Use	Abuse Potential
I	Heroin, LSD, hashish, marijuana, methaqualone, designer drugs	Unpredictable side effects, severe psychological or physical dependence, or death	No accepted use; some are legal for limited research only	Highest
II	Morphine, PCP, codeine, cocaine, methadone, Demerol®, benzedrine, dexedrine	May lead to severe psychological or physical dependence	Accepted use with restrictions	High
III	Codeine with aspirin or Tylenol®, some amphetamines, anabolic steroids	May lead to moderate or low physical dependence or high psychological dependence	Accepted use	Medium
IV	Darvon®, Talwin®, phenobarbital, Equanil®, Miltown®, Librium®, diazepam	May lead to limited physical or psychological dependence	Accepted use	Low
V	Over-the-counter or prescription compounds with codeine, Lomotil®, Robitussin AC®	May lead to limited physical or psychological dependence	Accepted use	Lowest

Comments This schedule of ranking specific drugs was derived by the Drug Enforcement Administration (DEA) as specified in the Controlled Substances Act. This ranking shows how potent, useful, and prone to abuse specific drugs are. It is also used to set benchmarks for determining penalties regarding drug abuse and trafficking. A Schedule I drug is the most strictly controlled, while a Schedule V drug is in the least severely regulated category.

Any person or organization can petition the DEA to "schedule" or rank a drug. The DEA conducts an initial evaluation and forwards its observations to the Department of Health and Human Services (HHS), which returns its recommendation to the DEA. If HHS recommends against scheduling a drug, the DEA cannot schedule it. If HHS recommends scheduling, the DEA must make a final determination to decide in which of the five categories the drug will be placed.

States also enact laws that schedule controlled substances and set penalties. Many state schedules are similar to the federal schedule. However, some drugs may be in different categories and some categories may be defined differently. The most common occurence of such a difference is with marijuana. Although it is a Schedule I drug on the federal list, most states create a separate category for it or leave it in the most severe category, but specify less severe penalties.

Source U.S. Department of Justice. Office of Justice Programs. Bureau of Justice Statistics. *Drugs, Crime, and the Justice System, A National Report from the Bureau of Justice Statistics, December 1992, NCJ-133652.* Washington, D.C.: U.S. Government Printing Office, [1992], p. 99. Primary source: Drug Enforcement Administration, *Drugs of Abuse:1989.*

Contact Drug Enforcement Administration, 600-700 Army Navy Dr., Arlington, VA 22202. Public Affairs: (202) 307-7977.

National Clearinghouse for Alcohol and Drug Information: (800) 729-6686.

Drug Use by Arrested Persons: 1991

Percentage of persons arrested in 24 U.S. cities, by gender, who tested positive
for a particular drug at the time of their arrest.

City	Male Arrestees, percent				Female Arrestees, percent			
	Any Drug	Mari-juana	Cocaine	Heroin	Any Drug	Mari-juana	Cocaine	Heroin
Atlanta, GA	63	12	57	3	70	8	66	4
Birmingham, AL	63	16	52	5	62	10	44	11
Chicago, IL	74	23	61	21	—	—	—	—
Cleveland, OH	56	12	48	3	79	7	76	6
Dallas, TX	56	19	43	4	56	11	45	9
Denver, CO	50	25	30	2	54	16	41	2
Detroit, MI	55	18	41	8	68	4	62	11
Fort Lauderdale, FL	61	28	44	1	64	14	55	4
Houston, TX	65	17	56	3	59	8	52	4
Indianapolis, IN	45	23	22	3	54	22	26	11
Kansas City, MO	53	18	37	1	64	13	56	4
Los Angeles, CA	62	19	44	10	75	9	62	18
Manhattan, NY	73	18	62	14	77	11	66	21
Miami, FL	68	23	61	2	—	—	—	—
New Orleans, LA	59	16	50	4	50	7	42	7
Omaha, NE	36	26	14	2	—	—	—	—
Philadelphia, PA	74	18	62	11	75	14	64	9
Phoenix, AZ	42	22	20	5	61	14	45	17
Portland, OR	61	33	30	9	68	28	40	17
St. Louis, MO	59	16	48	6	54	8	47	7
San Antonio, TX	49	20	31	16	45	9	25	21
San Diego, CA	75	33	45	17	73	20	40	21
San Jose, CA	58	25	33	8	52	13	30	7
Washington, DC	59	11	49	10	75	6	68	16

Comments Drug use by arrestees is measured through the Drug Use Forecasting (DUF) program sponsored by the National Institute of Justice. The data from the DUF program are collected in central booking facilities in participating cities throughout the U.S.

For about fourteen consecutive nights each quarter, trained local staff collect voluntary and anonymous urine specimens and interviews from a new sample group of arrestees (Chicago, Miami, and Omaha did not test or interview female arrestees). The category "any drug" includes cocaine, opiates, marijuana, phencyclidine (PCP), methadone, ben-zodiazepine, methaqualone, propoxyphene, barbiturates, and amphetamines.

Drug use differs not only by drug type, but also by city. (Certain drugs are more/less popular in certain cities, according to persons arrested who test positive for drugs.) For example, of the males tested for drugs in 1991, the percentages ranged from 36% (Omaha) to 75% (San Diego), while the range for females varied between 45% (San Antonio) and 77% (Manhattan). What can be inferred from this data is that some cities have a greater proportion of persons arrested who use drugs than do others.

Source U.S. Department of Justice. Office of Justice Programs. Bureau of Justice Statistics. *Sourcebook of Criminal Justice Statistics—1992,* Kathleen Maguire, Ann L. Pastore, and Timothy J. Flanagan, eds. Washington, D.C.: U. S. Government Printing Office, [1993], table 4.32, p. 459. Primary source: U.S. Department of Justice, National Institute of Justice, *Drug Use Forecasting 1991 Annual Report, NCJ-137776,* 1992, pp. 5, 7–9.

Contact Bureau of Justice Statistics Clearinghouse, Box 6000, Rockville, MD 20850; (800) 732-3277. Drugs & Crime Data Center & Clearinghouse, 1600 Research Blvd., Rockville, MD 20850; (800) 666-3332.

Sampling of Past Month Drug Use: 1992

Estimated use of illegal drugs in general, of marijuana, and cocaine
during the past month (at time of survey), by sex and age group.

Estimated use of any illicit drug in the past month

Age group	Male	Female	Total
12 to 17 years	5.7	6.5	6.1
18 to 25 years	16.7	9.5	13.0
26 to 34 years	12.6	7.6	10.1
35 years and older	3.2	1.4	2.2
Total all ages	7.1	4.1	5.5

Estimated use of marijuana during the past month

Age group	Male	Female	Total
12 to 17 years	4.6	3.5	4.0
18 to 25 years	14.5	7.5	11.0
26 to 34 years	11.0	5.5	8.2
35 years and older	2.3	1.0	1.6
Total all ages	5.9	2.9	4.4

Estimated use of cocaine during the past month

Age group	Male	Female	Total
12 to 17 years	0.2	0.3	0.3
18 to 25 years	2.9	0.8	1.8
26 to 34 years	1.7	1.1	1.4
35 years and older	0.3	0.1	0.2
Total all ages	0.9	0.4	0.6

Comments According to these estimates from a nationwide household survey in 1992 using random sampling, men were more likely than women to have used illicit drugs within the past month. This is particularly true for men between the ages of 18 and 25 years.

Among the 18 to 25 age group for men, the ratio of users of marijuana specifically was about two males to every female. For cocaine, however, the ratio was nearly three male users to every female user. For the 26 to 34 age group, there were also about two male users of marijuana for every female user, but the ratio of male to female cocaine users is less than two to one. Whereas cocaine use among men peaks between the ages of 18 and 25 years, it is most common among women aged 26 to 34 years.

Among adolescents aged 12 to 17, the use of any drug was more prevalent among females than males; differences for specific rates of marijuana and cocaine use between males and females were not as large as the 18 to 25 age group.

Source U.S. Department of Justice. Office of Justice Programs. Bureau of Justice Statistics. *Sourcebook of Criminal Justice Statistics—1992,* Kathleen Maguire, Ann L. Pastore, and Timothy J. Flanagan, eds. Washington, D.C.: U. S. Government Printing Office, [1993], pp. 342–344. Primary source: U.S. Department of Health and Human Services, Substance Abuse and Mental Health Services Administration, *Preliminary Estimates from the 1992 National Household Survey on Drug Abuse,* 1993, pp. 51, 53, 55.

Contact U.S. Department of Health and Human Services, Public Health Service, Substance Abuse and Mental Health Services Administration, National Institute on Drug Abuse, 5600 Fishers Lane, Rockville, MD 20857; (301) 443-6487. Public Relations: (301) 443-1124. National Clearinghouse for Alcohol and Drug Information: (800) 729-6686.

Liquor and Marijuana Use Among Youth and their Role in Violent Behavior: 1993–94

Comparison of the violent behavior of students who use marijuana and liquor with the violent behavior of those who do not. The subjects surveyed are 6th–8th graders and 9th–12 graders.

Behavior	% Using Liquor	% Using Marijuana	% Never Using Liquor	% Never Using Marijuana
6th–8th Graders				
Carrying a gun to school	66.6	56.2	19.0	6.2
Taking part in gang activities	52.0	31.9	15.7	4.3
Thinking of suicide often/a lot*	51.6	29.9	18.8	6.8
Threatening to harm another person	40.5	19.8	12.4	3.3
Getting in trouble with police	47.2	28.2	14.0	3.1
9th–12th Graders				
Carrying a gun to school	80.2	66.2	48.6	21.5
Taking part in gang activities	77.2	57.2	46.7	19.6
Thinking of suicide often/a lot*	73.0	49.8	49.1	22.8
Threatening to harm another person	69.5	41.9	41.0	15.6
Getting in trouble with police	75.3	51.8	41.9	14.8

* For "Thinking of suicide often/a lot," the responses are never, seldom, and some.

Comments

High school and junior high students who use marijuana seem to be much more likely to engage in certain types of violent behavior, according to the 1993–94 PRIDE USA Survey.

Students who bring guns to school, participate in gang activities, threaten a teacher or student, think about suicide, or get into trouble with the police are more likely to use drugs than are students who do not engage in these violent behaviors.

According to the survey, 4.3% of junior high school students and 7.4% of high school students reported having carried guns to school. Among the 6th–8th graders who had carried a gun to school, 56.2% reported using marijuana, while 6.2% reported never using marijuana. Among high school students who had carried guns to school, 66.2% reported using marijuana, while 21.5% reported never using marijuana.

This survey helps show the relationship between drug use and violence. Some violent behavior seems to follow drug use. This could mean that an increase in drug use may result in an increase in violent behavior. The quantity of drugs used could be related to violent behavior.

Source

Office of National Drug Control Policy. Executive Office of the President of the United States. *National Drug Control Strategy, Strengthening Communities' Response to Drugs and Crime, February 1995*. Washington, D.C.: U.S. Government Printing Office, [1995], pp. 31–32. Primary source: Parent Resource Institute for Drug Education, *1993–94 PRIDE USA Survey.*

Contact

National Parents' Resource Institute for Drug Education (PRIDE), 50 Hurt Plaza, Suite 210, Atlanta, GA 30303; (404) 577-4500. Executive Office of the President of the United States, Office of National Drug Control Policy, Washington, D.C. 20500; (202) 395-6700.

Young Adults' Past Month Drug Use: 1974–91

Trends in drug use in the past month (at time of survey)
by persons aged 18–25, in percent.

	1974	1976	1977	1979	1982	1985	1988	1990	1991
Any illicit drug	*	*	*	37	30	26	18	15	15
Marijuana or hashish	25	25	27	35	27	22	16	13	13
Inhalants	*	1	*	1	*	1	2	1	2
Hallucinogens	3	1	2	4	2	2	2	1	1
Cocaine	3	2	4	9	7	8	5	2	2
Nonmedical use of any psychotherapeutics	*	*	*	6	7	6	4	3	3
Stimulants	4	5	3	4	5	4	2	1	1
Sedatives	2	2	3	3	3	2	1	1	1
Tranquilizers	1	3	2	2	2	2	1	1	1
Analgesics	*	*	*	1	1	2	2	1	2

* This survey either did not include a question about that drug, or an estimate was not made for the category.

Comments Drug use by young adults has generally decreased since the late 1970s, as is shown by survey data presented here. However, declining rates may just be the result of an increasing reluctance of some to report drug use. Surveys can sometimes miss important segments of the population, which may lead to a difference between a survey's findings and actual conditions.

The age group examined here includes members of the household population, high school seniors, college athletes, and military personnel. The term "any illicit drug" refers to marijuana, hashish, cocaine (including crack), inhalants, hallucinogens (including PCP), heroin, or nonmedical use of psychotherapeutics used at least once. Heroin use in the past month in this survey was too low to use for a national estimate.

This survey presents the number of young adults who use drugs within a given month, but it does not report frequently drugs were used within that month.

Source U.S. Department of Justice. Office of Justice Programs. Bureau of Justice Statistics. *Drugs, Crime, and the Justice System, A National Report from the Bureau of Justice Statistics, December 1992, NCJ-133652.* Washington, D.C.: U.S. Government Printing Office, [1992], p. 31. Primary source: National Institute on Drug Abuse, *National Household Survey on Drug Abuse: Main Findings, 1990*, 1991, table 2.11; and *National Household Survey on Drug Abuse: Population Estimates, 1991*, 1991.

Contact U.S. Department of Health and Human Services, Public Health Service, Substance Abuse and Mental Health Services Administration, National Institute on Drug Abuse, 5600 Fishers Lane, Rockville, MD 20857; (301) 443-6487. Public Relations: (301) 443-1124. National Clearinghouse for Alcohol and Drug Information: (800) 729-6686.

Steroid Use by High School Seniors: 1989–94

Percentage of high school seniors using steroids, reported by frequency of use.

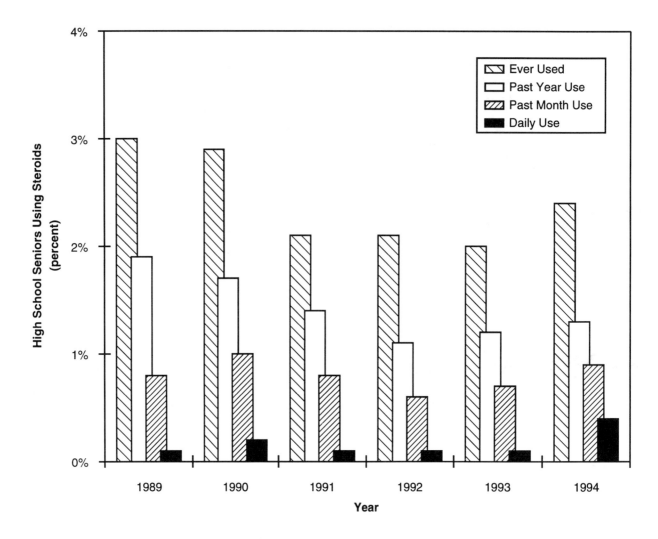

	1989	1990	1991	1992	1993	1994
Ever used	3.0	2.9	2.1	2.1	2.0	2.4
Past year use	1.9	1.7	1.4	1.1	1.2	1.3
Past month use	0.8	1.0	0.8	0.6	0.7	0.9
Daily use	0.1	0.2	0.1	0.1	0.1	0.4

Comments   Unlike most illicit drug use, steroid use is prompted by a different motive. Rather than mental euphoria, excitement, or relaxation, the desired effects of steroids on users (usually anabolic steroids) are physical rather than mental.

Anabolic steroids are synthetic hormones that are used to increase the body's metabolism. The use of steroids temporarily increases muscle mass, which is often perceived as a competitive advantage by athletes (especially in sports where body size and strength are crucial, like football and wrestling). The induced metabolic increase through continued steroid use, however, can result in serious health complications that have been fatal in some cases. Because the desired effect is different from most illicit drugs, steroid users may not be inclined to use any other drug. They may even abstain from using alcohol and tobacco, which are typically consumed by psychotropic drug users.

Source   U.S. Department of Health and Human Services. Public Health Service. Substance Abuse and Mental Health Services Administration. National Institute on Drug Abuse. *Monitoring the Future Study, 1975–1994: National High School Senior Drug Abuse Survey,* 1994, pp. 2–5.

Contact   U.S. Department of Health and Human Services, Public Health Service, Substance Abuse and Mental Health Services Administration, National Institute on Drug Abuse, 5600 Fishers Lane, Rockville, MD 20857; (301) 443-6487. Public Relations: (301) 443-1124. National Clearinghouse for Alcohol and Drug Information: (800) 729-6686.

Drug Use by U.S. Military Personnel: 1992

Percent of military personnel using drugs, reported by the type of drug, branch of service, and most recent use at time of survey.

Drug	U.S. Department of Defense Total		Army		Navy		Marine Corps		Air Force	
	Past 30 Days	Past 12 Months	Past 30 Days	Past 12 Months	Past 30 Days	Past 12 Months	Past 30 Days	Past 12 Months	Past 30 Days	Past 12 Months
Marijuana	1.5	3.8	1.8	5.1	1.8	3.8	3.0	7.8	0.3	0.8
Cocaine	0.7	1.7	0.8	2.1	1.1	2.5	0.6	2.0	0.1	0.2
PCP	0.0	0.3	0.0	0.2	0.1	0.4	0.0	0.5	0.1	0.1
LSD/ hallucinogens	0.9	1.8	0.8	1.8	1.3	2.4	2.2	4.0	0.1	0.2
Amphetamines/ stimulants	0.3	0.7	0.4	0.9	0.2	0.9	0.5	0.8	0.2	0.2
Tranquilizers	0.3	0.6	0.4	0.9	0.2	0.4	0.4	0.8	0.2	0.3
Barbiturates/ sedatives	0.1	0.3	0.2	0.5	0.2	0.3	0.0	0.3	0.1	0.1
Heroin/other opiates	0.0	0.2	0.0	0.1	0.1	0.1	0.0	0.8	0.1	0.1
Analgesics	1.1	1.5	1.0	1.5	1.3	1.8	1.5	1.9	0.7	1.0
Inhalants	0.5	0.6	0.7	0.8	0.7	0.9	0.3	0.5	0.2	0.2
Designer drugs	0.3	0.5	0.2	0.6	0.5	0.6	0.5	0.8	0.1	0.1
Any drug*	3.4	6.2	3.9	7.7	4.0	6.6	5.6	10.7	1.2	2.3
Any drug except marijuana†	2.6	4.5	3.1	5.4	3.1	5.5	3.9	6.9	1.0	1.7
Anabolic steroids	0.2	0.3	0.1	0.5	0.1	0.1	0.6	0.9	0.2	0.2

* Nonmedical use one or more times of any drug(s) listed in the table except steroids.

† Nonmedical use one or more times of any drug(s) listed in the table except marijuana and steroids.

Comments Under the direction of the Department of Defense, the Research Triangle Institute conducted a series of surveys of military personnel in 1980, 1982, 1985, 1988, and 1992.

The populations of these surveys include all active-duty military personnel except recruits, service academy students, persons absent without leave, and persons who had a permanent change of station at the time of data collection. The sampling for these surveys took into account differences in geographic location and pay grade to represent a wide diversity of military personnel. According to the 1992 survey, drug use was generally lowest in the air force, while highest in the marine corps.

Marijuana was the most commonly used drug in all military branches; analgesics also were among the most frequently used drugs. The use of cocaine and inhalants was higher in the army and navy than in the marine corps and air force. Tranquilizers were more commonly used by persons either in the army or marine corps. Anabolic steroids (taken for temporary muscle enhancement rather than for mind-altering effects) were most likely to have been used by marine corps personnel.

Source U.S. Department of Justice. Office of Justice Programs. Bureau of Justice Statistics. *Sourcebook of Criminal Justice Statistics—1992,* Kathleen Maguire, Ann L. Pastore, and Timothy J. Flanagan, eds. Washington, D.C.: U. S. Government Printing Office, [1993], table 3.94, p. 335. Primary source: Robert M. Bray, et. al., *1992 Worldwide Survey of Substance Abuse and Health Behaviors Among Military Personnel,* 1992, pp.5–12.

Contact Research Triangle Institute, 3040 Cornwallis Rd., P.O. Box 12194, Research Triangle Park, NC 27709; (919) 541-6000.

Drugs & Crime Data Center & Clearinghouse, 1600 Research Blvd., Rockville, MD 20850; (800) 666-3332.

Drug Testing Programs in Private Business: 1989

Percent of private establishments in a given industry with drug testing programs for employees and applicants for employment.

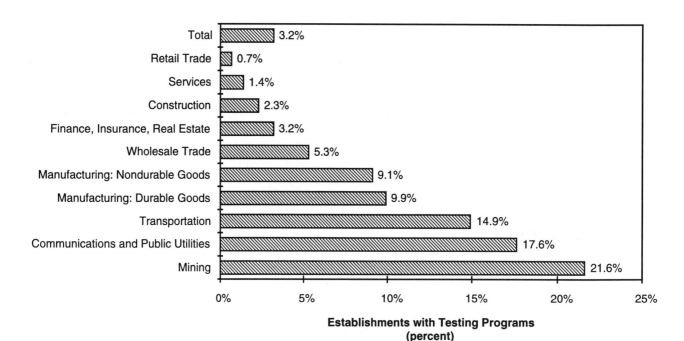

Establishments with Testing Programs
(percent)

	Percent of Establishments with Testing Programs	Total Number of Establishments in Industry
Mining	21.6	31,600
Communications and public utilities	17.6	37,500
Transportation	14.9	153,500
Manufacturing: Durable goods	9.9	193,900
Manufacturing: Nondurable goods	9.1	141,200
Wholesale trade	5.3	467,900
Finance, insurance, real estate	3.2	403,900
Construction	2.3	458,100
Services	1.4	1,553,400
Retail trade	0.7	1,101,800
TOTAL	3.2	4,542,800

Comments Drug testing is an approach used by employers to detect drug use. Drug use by an employee can impair coordination and decision-making. Either effect could decrease safety and/or efficiency in the workplace. In industries where the public relies heavily upon the composure of an individual, drug use by an employee can impose a serious threat. (Examples of such employees are transportation workers and armed security guards).

In regulated industries like defense contracting, nuclear energy, and transportation, a large number of public and private employees are subject to periodic drug tests. For example, the Department of Transportation requires public and private industries that it regulates to use five types of drug tests: pre-employment, periodic (as part of required medical exams), random, reasonable cause, and post-accident.

Large businesses are more likely to have drug testing programs than smaller ones (43% of the 5,600 businesses with more than 1,000 employees versus 2% of the 4.2 million with fewer than 50).

According to this survey, relatively few workers for private businesses are actually tested. Only about 1% of all workers and 4 million applicants were tested in the year before the information presented here was collected.

About 9% of employee and 12% of applicant test results were positive. However, the Bureau of Labor Statistics has noted that these results cannot be applied to the entire work force, since such a small proportion of workers were tested, and many of them were tested because of suspected drug use.

Source U.S. Department of Justice. Office of Justice Programs. Bureau of Justice Statistics. *Drugs, Crime, and the Justice System, A National Report from the Bureau of Justice Statistics, December 1992, NCJ-* *133652.* Washington, D.C.: U.S. Government Printing Office, [1992], p.116. Primary source: Bureau of Labor Statistics, *Survey of Employer Anti-Drug Programs,* January 1989, table 2.

Contact U.S. Department of Labor, Bureau of Labor Statistics, Office of Safety, Health and Working Conditions, 2 Massachusetts Ave. NE, Washington, D.C. 20212; (202) 606-6304.

Deaths in the Workplace Involving Drugs: 1992

Fatal injuries on the job listed by type of accident or exposure to harmful substances, reported by type of drug detected in fatally injured worker. The totals shown here were taken from 1,355 detailed death reports. Those 1,355 reports represented only 25% of all job-related deaths in 1992.

	Cocaine	Marijuana	Other Drugs**	Alcohol	Total Drugs and Alcohol*
Highway incidents	9	—	6	18	35
Other transportation incidents	—	4	—	17	25
Harmful exposures	8	7	8	15	38
Falls	4	6	5	10	25
Contact with object	—	6	—	9	18
Fires and explosions	—	—	—	—	3
Homicide	10	—	9	25	45
Suicide	—	—	4	14	19
TOTAL*	36	27	36	112	211

* Numbers do not add because some cases were counted more than once.
** Includes antidepressants, amphetamines, barbiturates, morphine, codeine, and methadone.

These statistics provide insight into the relationship between drug use and fatal injuries in the workplace.

In 1992, there were 6,083 job-related deaths across the U.S. The Bureau of Labor Statistics' Census of Fatal Occupational Injuries (CFOI) program collected 1,355 toxicology reports from 43 states and the District of Columbia. These states and the District of Columbia had 5,444 fatal occupational injuries.

It is important to remember that the statistics shown here only represent about 25% of the 5,444 fatal occupational injuries occurring in these jurisdictions during 1992. Of the 1,355 toxicology reports submitted, about one-sixth were positive for some toxic substance (e.g., drugs, alcohol, carbon monoxide). Using this fraction, it is possible to estimate the total involvement of alcohol and drugs in job-related deaths. If one-sixth of the 6,083 job-related deaths involved drugs or alcohol, then over 1,000 people died on the job in 1992 due to the effects of drugs or alcohol. After alcohol, cocaine was the second most frequently identified substance and was detected in 19% of intentional deaths (homicide and suicide) and 15% of unintentional deaths.

Some of the rows and columns of numbers given in the chart do not add up to the total given because some cases were counted in more than one category. For example, if one of the toxicology reports had been positive for cocaine and alcohol, one mention for each would occur under those categories, even though the cocaine and alcohol were detected in the same person.

According to the CFOI report, the use of alcohol and drugs made an indirect but critical contribution to the large majority of deaths associated with toxic substances. Most workers were accidentally killed due to the effects of the drug(s) on mental perception or physical coordination rather than by the use of the drug itself.

The only available information was about the victims and not the perpetrators. Therefore, the role of drugs in work-related homicides cannot be fully understood by these statistics.

Source U.S. Department of Labor. Bureau of Labor Statistics. *Census of Fatal Occupational Injuries, 1992*. U.S. Department of Labor, Bureau of Labor Statistics. William

M. Marine, M.D. and Tracy Jack, "Analysis of Toxicology Reports from the 1992 Census of Fatal Occupational Injuries," *Compensation and Working Conditions*, October 1994.

Contact U.S. Department of Labor, Bureau of Labor Statistics, Office of Safety, Health and Working Conditions, 2 Massachusetts Ave. NE, Washington, D.C. 20212; (202) 606-6304.

Drug-Related Murders in the U.S.: 1986–93

The relationship between drug-related murders and the total of all murders in the U.S.

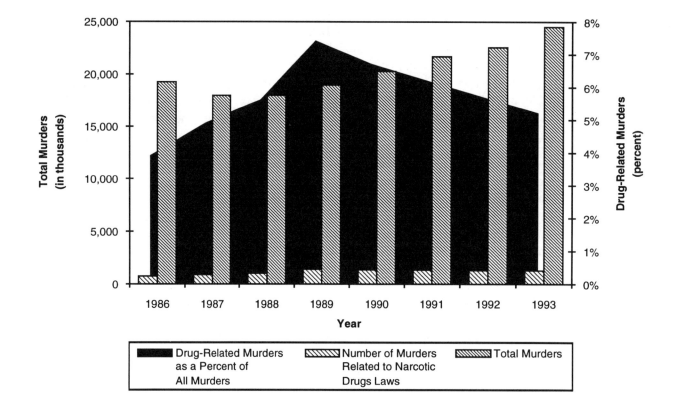

Year	Total Murders	Murders Related to Narcotic Drugs Laws	Drug-Related Murders as a Percent of All Murders
1986	19,257	751	3.9%
1987	17,963	880	4.9%
1988	17,971	1,006	5.6%
1989	18,954	1,403	7.4%
1990	20,273	1,358	6.7%
1991	21,676	1,344	6.2%
1992	22,540	1,285	5.7%
1993	24,526	1,287	5.2%

Comments   This bar chart illustrates the relationship between drug-related murders and all murders in the U.S. from 1986 to 1993. Nationally, drug-related murders as a percent of all murders rose steadily in the mid-1980s, peaking at 7.4% in 1989, before falling back to 5.2% in 1993. These statistics, however, do not necessarily include murders where drugs were a motivational factor (e.g., murders committed during an armed robbery for money to maintain a drug addiction). These numbers also fail to state that according to a recent study between 1985 and 1992 the number of homicides committed by youths ages 18 and younger more than doubled, while there has been no growth in homicide rates by adults aged 24 and older. (*Youth, Violence, and the Illicit Drug Industry*, by A. Blumstein, from the H. John Heinz II School of Public Policy and Management, Working Paper Series, July 1994.)

Source   Office of National Drug Control Policy. Executive Office of the President of the United States. *National Drug Control Strategy, Strengthening Communities' Response to Drugs and Crime, February 1995*. Washington, D.C.: U.S. Government Printing Office, [1995], pp. 29–30. Primary source: Bureau of Justice Statistics, *Drug and Crime Facts, 1993–94.*

Contact   Bureau of Justice Statistics Clearinghouse, Box 6000, Rockville, MD 20850; (800) 732-3277. Drugs & Crime Data Center & Clearinghouse, 1600 Research Blvd., Rockville, MD 20850, (800) 666-3332.

THC Content of Seized Marijuana: 1975–90

Potency of types of marijuana according to percent of THC (chemical producing euphoric effect).

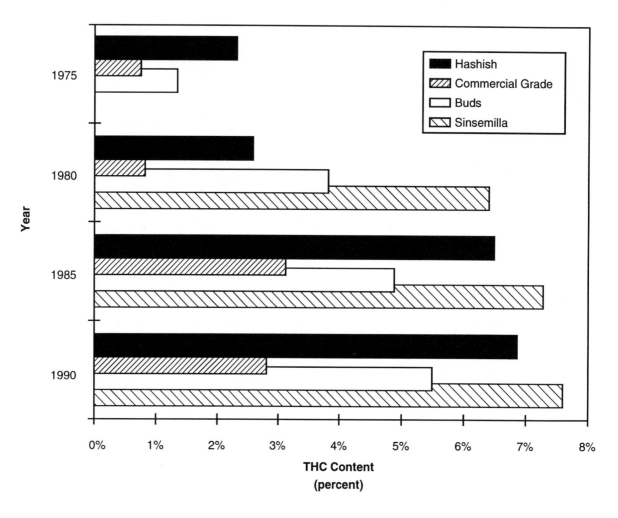

	1975	1980	1985	1990
Sinsemilla	—	6.40	7.28	7.60
Buds	1.34	3.81	4.88	5.49
Commercial grade	0.75	0.82	3.12	2.81
Hashish	2.31	2.58	6.49	6.86

Comments Tetrahydrocannabinol (THC) is the chemical substance within marijuana that produces the desired euphoric effect for drug users. Drug dealers and traffickers have sought to make their product more potent to satisfy their customers' demand for greater highs. Moreover, the more potent the drug, the smaller its size becomes relative to its value, making it less costly to transport and easier to smuggle.

The various grades of marijuana differ widely in THC potency. For example, the sinsemilla (a term coined from Spanish, meaning "without seed") type comes from female plants that are specifically grown and kept from pollinating and therefore from producing seeds. This produces more THC-rich resin within the plant. The flowering buds of the plant are themselves rich in THC and are often sold exclusively; commercial grade consists of the ordinary leaves (perhaps with some stems or seeds mixed in).

Hashish, produced mainly in the Middle East, comes from the THC-rich resin of the cannabis plant which is dried and compressed into balls or sheets. The hashish is produced by repeatedly extracting the plant materials until only a dark oily liquid is left. Hashish users make up only a very small portion of the marijuana user population of the U.S. This may be because users prefer domestically grown marijuana with a high THC content or are unfamiliar with the product.

Source U.S. Department of Justice Office of Justice Programs. Bureau of Justice Statistics. *Drugs, Crime, and the Justice System, A National Report from the Bureau of Justice Statistics, December 1992, NCJ-133652.* Washington, D.C.: U.S. Government Printing Office, [1992], p. 53. Primary source: National Narcotics Intelligence Consumers Committee, *The NNICC Report 1990: The Supply of Illicit Drugs to the United States,* June 1991, p. 30.

Contact Bureau of Justice Statistics Clearinghouse, Box 6000, Rockville, MD 20850; (800) 732-3277. Drugs & Crime Data Center & Clearinghouse, 1600 Research Blvd., Rockville, MD 20850; (800) 666-3332.

Drug-Related Arrests: 1988–93

Percent of all arrests in the U.S. which are drug related.

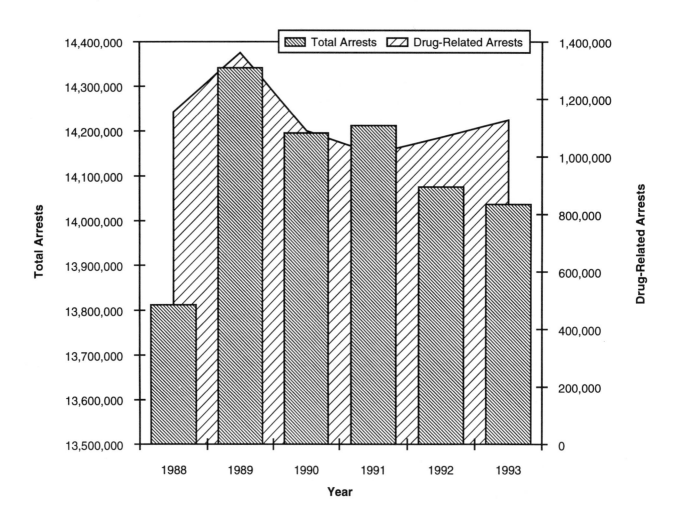

	1988	1989	1990	1991	1992	1993
Total arrests	13,812,300	14,340,900	14,195,100	14,211,900	14,075,100	14,036,300
Drug-related arrests	1,155,200	1,361,700	1,089,500	1,010,000	1,066,400	1,126,300
Percent of all arrests which are drug related	8.4%	9.5%	7.7%	7.1%	7.6%	8.0%

Comments The FBI reported over 1.1 million arrests for drug law violations in 1993. This was down from the peak of 1989, but still the second highest ever recorded. These drug law offenders have created an enormous strain on the criminal justice system and in some instances have taken prison space needed for violent offenders. According to the Bureau of Justice Statistics, the federal and state prison population in 1994 exceeded one million inmates for the first time in U.S. history; this growth in recent years is largely attributable to the rise in the number of persons arrested for drug law violations. The number of persons arrested for drug law violations also reflects more severe drug laws, especially in the area of mandatory minimum sentences.

Source Office of National Drug Control Policy. Executive Office of the President of the United States. *National Drug Control Strategy, Strengthening Communities' Response to Drugs and Crime, February 1995.* Washington, D.C.: U.S. Government Printing Office, [1995], p. 35. Primary source: Federal Bureau of Investigation, National Uniform Crime Reporting Program, 1988–93.

Contact Uniform Crime Reports, Criminal Justice Information Services Division, FBI/GRB, Washington, D.C. 20535. Information Dissemination: (202) 324-5015.

Drug Use During Crimes: 1990

Percent of persons by gender who tested positive for any drug after arrest for selected crimes.

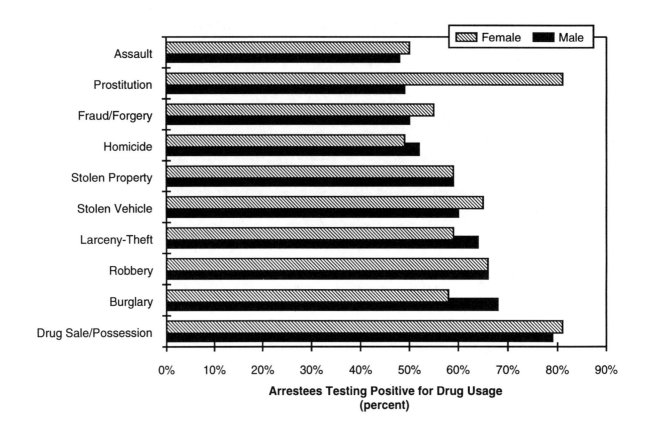

**Arrestees Testing Positive for Drug Usage
(percent)**

Crime	Male	Female
Drug sale/possession	79	81
Burglary	68	58
Robbery	66	66
Larceny-theft	64	59
Stolen vehicle	60	65
Stolen property	59	59
Homicide	52	49
Fraud/forgery	50	55
Prostitution	49	81
Assault	48	50

Comments

In 1990, the Drug Use Forecasting Program (DUF) gathered voluntary urinalysis results from 19,883 male arrestees in 23 cities, and 7,947 female arrestees in 21 cities. The urinalysis tested for use of drugs including cocaine, opiates, PCP, marijuana, amphetamines, methadone, methaqualone, benzodiazepines, barbiturates, and propoxyphene. The DUF reported that 60% or more of the males arrested that year for property crimes (burglary, larceny-theft, stolen vehicles) and for robbery were found to be positive for drug use, as were 50% or more of the females arrested for burglary, robbery, and stolen vehicles.

Some crimes, like drug sale/possession and burglary had a higher number of arrestees testing positive for drugs than did crimes such as assault or fraud/forgery. Some crimes, like larceny-theft, had a greater share of male arrestees testing positive for drugs. The proportion of women arrested for prostitution who tested positive was vastly greater than the percentage of male arrestees for prostitution with a positive drug test.

Many illegal drugs—like heroin and cocaine—are expensive as well as addictive. In order to purchase drugs, some users commit property crimes like burglary, larceny-theft, motor vehicle theft, forgery, fraud, arson, dealing in stolen property, and embezzlement. Robbery can also bring in quick cash but is typically considered a violent crime since it involves the use or threat of force. Other crimes sometimes committed for money to support a drug habit include prostitution and drug trafficking. Disputes and/or blackmail stemming from these crimes sometimes results in violence.

Source

U.S. Department of Justice. Office of Justice Programs. Bureau of Justice Statistics. *Drugs, Crime, and the Justice System, A National Report from the Bureau of Justice Statistics, December 1992, NCJ-133652*. Washington, D.C.: U.S. Government Printing Office, [1992], p. 7. Primary source: National Institute of Justice, 1990 Drug Use Forecasting Program, unpublished data.

Contact

Bureau of Justice Statistics Clearinghouse, Box 6000, Rockville, MD 20850; (800) 732-3277. Drugs & Crime Data Center & Clearinghouse, 1600 Research Blvd., Rockville, MD 20850, (800) 666-3332.

Regional Distribution of Drug Law Violation Arrests: 1981–1993

Comparison of proportion of arrests in four regions of the U.S. by type of drug law violation.

Year	Total U.S. Sale/Manufacture	Posses-sion	Northeast Sale/Manufacture	Posses-sion	Midwest Sale/Manufacture	Posses-sion	South Sale/Manufacture	Posses-sion	West Sale/Manufacture	Posses-sion
1981	22	78	22	78	33	67	20	80	16	84
1982	20	80	24	76	22	78	21	79	13	87
1983	22	78	27	73	24	76	24	76	16	84
1984	22	78	30	70	24	76	21	79	15	85
1985	24	76	30	70	26	74	24	76	18	82
1986	25	75	33	67	26	74	25	75	19	81
1987	26	74	34	66	28	72	24	76	20	80
1988	27	73	35	65	31	69	27	73	21	79
1989	32	68	37	63	46	54	29	71	26	74
1990	32	68	41	59	32	68	28	72	28	72
1991	33	67	45	55	30	70	31	69	28	72
1992	32	68	43	57	30	70	29	71	27	73
1993	30	70	41	59	29	71	27	73	25	75

Comments These statistics highlight the proportions of drug law violations from the early 1980s to the early 1990s. They also show how the types of arrests vary by region of the country. "Sales and manufacturing" refer to drug trafficking, which can also involve distributing, dispensing, importing, or exporting a controlled substance. "Possession" refers to the illegal ownership of small amounts of a controlled substance for personal use. It is usually treated as a less serious crime, especially for a first-time offender.

The percentages of sale/manufacturing and possession arrestees added together account for all drug law violation arrestees for any of the given regions. Across the U.S., the proportion of arrestees for possession has gradually fallen since the early 1980s, with more emphasis placed on making arrests of individuals involved in the sale or manufacturing of illicit drugs. This focus represents a strategy to reduce the drug problem by disrupting supply. If manufacturers, distributors, and sellers of illicit drugs are arrested and possibly incarcerated, then (as the strategy follows) those who want to buy drugs will be inconvenienced—or unsuccessful—when trying to find a supply of drugs.

Among each of the four regions of the U.S., the changes in the percentages of arrestees for sale/manufacturing and possession since the early 1980s have varied. For instance, within the northeast and west, the proportion of sale/manufacturing arrests to possession arrests in the early 1990s has significantly increased since the early 1980s. In the midwest and south, the proportions have not changed as dramatically.

Source U.S. Department of Justice. Office of Justice Programs. Bureau of Justice Statistics. *Sourcebook of Criminal Justice Statistics—1992,* Kathleen Maguire, Ann L. Pastore, and Timothy J. Flanagan, eds. Washington, D.C.: U. S. Government Printing Office, [1993], table 4.30, p. 458. Primary source: U.S. Department of Justice, Federal Bureau of Investigation, *Crime in the United States, 1981*, p. 160; *1982*, p. 165; *1983*, p. 168; *1984*, p. 161; *1985*, p. 163; *1986*, p. 163; *1987*, p. 163; *1988*, p. 167; *1989*, p. 171; *1990*, p. 173; *1991*, p. 212; *1992*, p. 216; *1993*, p. 216.

Contact Bureau of Justice Statistics Clearinghouse, Box 6000, Rockville, MD 20850; (800) 732-3277. Drugs & Crime Data Center & Clearinghouse, 1600 Research Blvd., Rockville, MD 20850; (800) 666-3332. Uniform Crime Reports, Criminal Justice Information Services Division, FBI/GRB, Washington, D.C. 20535. Information Dissemination: (202) 324-5015.

How Drug Cases Are Handled: 1992

How drug cases are handled compared to other criminal offenses in the U.S. criminal justice system.

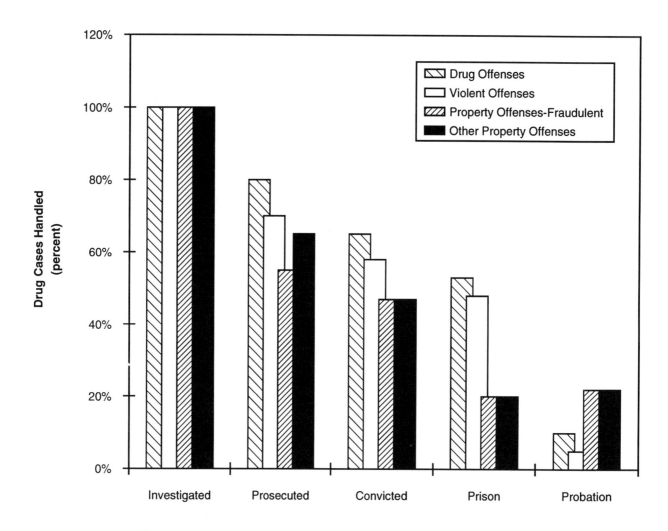

	Drug Offenses	Violent Offenses	Property Offenses– Fraudulent	Other Property Offenses
Investigated	100%	100%	100%	100%
Prosecuted	80%	70%	55%	65%
Convicted	65%	58%	47%	47%
Prison	53%	48%	20%	20%
Probation	10%	5%	22%	22%

Comments

Just because someone is investigated for a drug law violation does not necessarily mean that the individual will end up in prison. Like any criminal case subject to decision-making processes at different levels, drug cases drop out at various stages of the criminal justice system.

For example, prosecutors can decline to prosecute, file different charges from the arrest charges, or request dismissal of a case. Judges decide at the preliminary hearing if there is probable cause to believe that the accused committed a crime; grand juries determine if there is sufficient evidence to bring the accused to trial; and finally, judges and juries decide if an accused brought to trial is guilty beyond a reasonable doubt.

Most jurisdictions recognize two classes of offenses: felonies and misdemeanors. Generally, more serious drug offenses—such as selling large amounts of illegal drugs—are considered felonies. Less serious offenses—like possession of small amounts of marijuana—are misdemeanors. Most jurisdictions define felonies as offenses punishable by a year or more in prison.

"Investigated" drug cases represent a proportion of all potential drug cases, as many go undetected. According to the chart, however, of all the drug offense cases investigated (represented by 100%), over 80% will result in prosecution, over 60% of those investigated will be convicted, and over one-half of those investigated will receive prison sentences. The ratio of those receiving prison sentences for all investigated drug offenses is greater than the corresponding ratio for any other type of offense.

Source

U.S. Department of Justice. Office of Justice Programs. Bureau of Justice Statistics. *Drugs, Crime, and the Justice System, A National Report from the Bureau of Justice Statistics, December 1992, NCJ-133652.* Washington, D.C.: U.S. Government Printing Office, [1992], p.165. Primary source: Bureau of Justice Statistics, *Compendium of Federal Justice Statistics, 1989, NCJ-134730,* May 1992.

Contact

Bureau of Justice Statistics Clearinghouse, Box 6000, Rockville, MD 20850; (800) 732-3277. Drugs & Crime Data Center & Clearinghouse, 1600 Research Blvd., Rockville, MD 20850; (800) 666-3332.

Offenses for which Prisoners are Admitted to State Prisons: 1982–92

Trends in the categories of offenses for which sentenced prisoners are admitted to state prisons, by percent of admissions in each category.

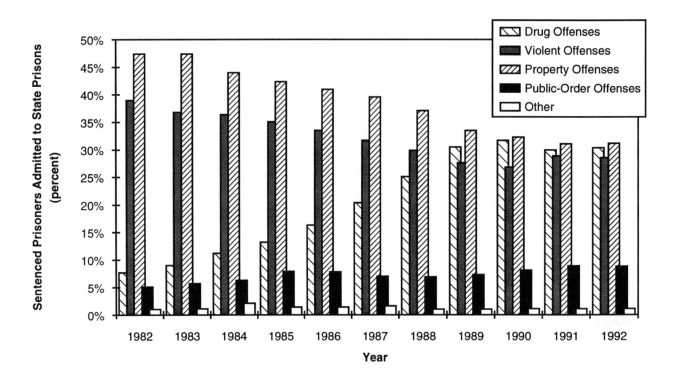

Year	Drug Offenses	Violent Offenses	Property Offenses	Public-Order Offenses	Other
1982	7.7%	39.0%	47.4%	5.1%	1.0%
1983	9.0%	36.8%	47.4%	5.7%	1.1%
1984	11.2%	36.4%	44.0%	6.3%	2.1%
1985	13.2%	35.1%	42.4%	7.9%	1.4%
1986	16.3%	33.5%	41.0%	7.8%	1.4%
1987	20.4%	31.7%	39.6%	7.0%	1.6%
1988	25.1%	29.9%	37.1%	6.9%	1.0%
1989	30.5%	27.6%	33.5%	7.3%	1.0%
1990	31.7%	26.8%	32.3%	8.1%	1.1%
1991	30.0%	28.9%	31.1%	8.9%	1.1%
1992	30.4%	28.6%	31.2%	8.8%	1.1%

Comments The accompanying statistics and chart illustrate percent changes for the offense category under which prisoners were sentenced to state prisons in the years shown. For instance, of all the state prisoners admitted in 1982, 7.7% were admitted for being convicted and sentenced for drug offenses, 39% for violent offenses, 47.4% for property offenses, etc. By 1990, the proportion of new state prisoner admissions for drug offenses had risen to 31.7%, while the percentages admitted for violent and property offenses shrank. These percentages, however, do not give any indication of the actual numbers of state prisoners admitted each year—they are only useful in examining the overall trend of reasons sentenced prisoners are admitted to state prisons. The use of percentages is an excellent tool for understanding the relationship between a part and the whole; however, percentages cannot give much give insight into changes in actual numerical values over time.

Source U.S. Department of Justice. Bureau of Justice Statistics. *Correctional Populations in the United States, 1992*, by Tracy L. Snell. Washington, D.C.: Bureau of Justice Statistics, January 1995, p. 57.

Contact Bureau of Justice Statistics Clearinghouse, Box 6000, Rockville, MD 20850; (800) 732-3277. Drugs & Crime Data Center & Clearinghouse, 1600 Research Blvd., Rockville, MD 20850; (800) 666-3332.

Inmates in State Prisons and Proportion of Drug Offenders: 1979–92

The estimated number and percentage of inmates in state prisons who are convicted drug offenders compared to estimated total number of state prisoners.

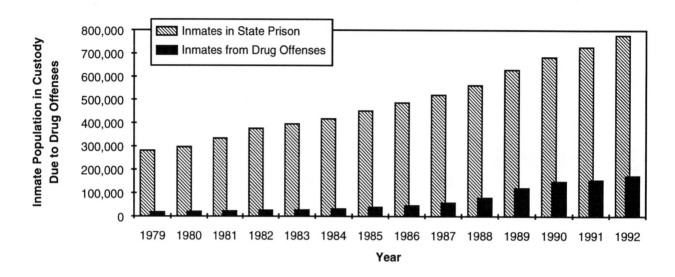

Year	Number of Inmates in State Prison	Inmates from Drug Offenses	As Percent of Inmates in State Prison
1979	281,233	18,000	6.4
1980	295,819	19,000	6.4
1981	333,251	21,700	6.5
1982	375,603	25,300	6.7
1983	394,953	26,600	6.7
1984	417,389	31,700	7.6
1985	451,812	38,900	8.6
1986	486,655	45,400	9.3
1987	520,336	57,900	11.1
1988	562,605	79,100	14.1
1989	629,995	120,100	19.1
1990	684,544	148,600	21.7
1991	728,605	155,200	21.3
1992	778,495	172,300	22.1

Comments This chart and table illustrate how the number of convicted drug offenders has increased as a proportion of state prison inmates since the mid-1980s. Since the data presented here include all state prisoners (inmates housed outside of state facilities are excluded), the turnover of prisoners from one year to the next cannot be addressed.

In order for a proportion of total inmates admitted for a drug offense to rise, however, many new convicted drug offenders would have to have been admitted during those years to offset those already in prison serving time for some other offense (e.g., violent, property, or public-order offenses). As the proportion of inmates serving time for a drug offense climbed, the proportions of inmates serving time for violent and property offenses dropped; the percentage of convicted public-order offenders remained fairly constant. These numbers, however, fail to show what role drugs may have had in other offenses for which prisoners have been sentenced. For instance, a prisoner may have been sentenced because of a violent or property crime related to drug use or trafficking.

Source Snell, Tracy L. *Correctional Populations in the United States, 1992.* Washington, D.C.: U.S. Department of Justice, Bureau of Justice Statistics, January 1995, p. 53–54.

Contact Bureau of Justice Statistics Clearinghouse, Box 6000, Rockville, MD 20850; (800) 732-3277. Drugs & Crime Data Center & Clearinghouse, 1600 Research Blvd., Rockville, MD 20850; (800) 666-3332.

Demographic Characteristics of Convicted Drug Felons: 1992

Convicted drug possession and trafficking felons and their demographic percentages as to race, gender, and age group.

		Possession	Trafficking
Gender	Male	83	86
	Female	17	14
Race	White	44	44
	Black	55	55
	Other	1	1
Age at sentencing	13–19	7	7
	20–29	42	49
	30–39	37	33
	40–49	12	9
	50–59	2	2
	60+		
	Average age	31	30
	Median age	30	28

Comments In 1992, there were an estimated 280,232 felonious drug offense convictions in state courts. These comprised 31.3% of all state court felony convictions. Possession felony convictions numbered an estimated 109,426 (12.2% of the total). Trafficking felony convictions amounted to about 170,806 (19.1%).

Men comprised nearly 50% of the adult U.S. population in 1992, but made up the overwhelming majority of possession and trafficking offense convictions that year. Similarly, whites were 86% of the U.S. adult population, but were 44% of persons convicted of a drug felony. Blacks were 11% of the U.S. adult population, but were 55% of convicted drug felons in 1992. The age category indicates that about half the convicted drug felons for both possession and trafficking in 1992 were in their 20s at the time of sentencing.

Since data for only one year are presented here, it is not possible to compare these findings with another year to make any general observations; without the presentation of data from other years, it is not possible to tell whether 1992 was a typical year or a total aberration.

Source U.S. Department of Justice. Office of Justice Programs. Bureau of Justice Statistics. *Felony Sentences in State Courts, 1992*. Washington, D.C.: U.S. Government Printing Office, January 1995, table 5, p. 5.

Contact Bureau of Justice Statistics Clearinghouse, Box 6000, Rockville, MD 20850; (800) 732-3277. Drugs & Crime Data Center & Clearinghouse, 1600 Research Blvd., Rockville, MD 20850; (800) 666-3332.

Average Lengths of Drug Felony Sentences: 1992

Average lengths (in months) of drug felony sentences imposed by state courts, according to the number of conviction offenses and type of felony.

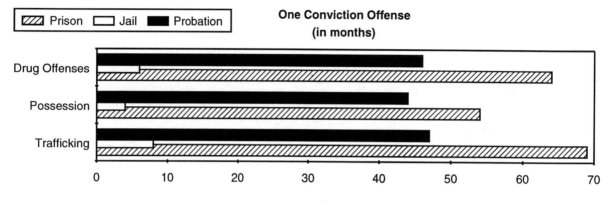

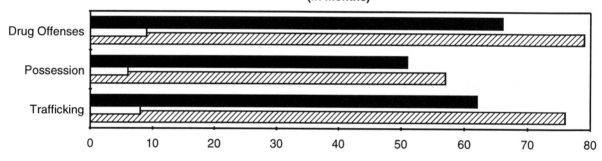

	Total	Prison	Jail	Probation (months)
One Conviction Offense				
Drug offenses	40	64	6	46
Possession	31	54	4	44
Trafficking	46	69	8	47
Two or More Conviction Offenses				
Drug offenses	54	76	8	62
Possession	37	57	6	51
Trafficking	58	79	9	66

Comments The punishment that a convicted drug felon receives depends on several factors. These include whether the offense was for possession or trafficking (with the former dealt with less harshly than the latter), the number of prior conviction offenses, and the way in which the sentence will be carried out (i.e., in a prison, a jail, or with probation). For example, sentences for possession were generally lighter than those for trafficking; felons with one conviction offense were given shorter sentences than those with two or more; probation sentences were longer than incarcerations; and when a felon was incarcerated, prison terms exceeded jail terms. A person with one conviction who is convicted of possession receives only about half the sentence that someone convicted of trafficking (with two or more convictions) receives.

Source U.S. Department of Justice. Office of Justice Programs. Bureau of Justice Statistics. *Felony Sentences in State Courts, 1992.* Washington, D.C.: U.S. Government Printing Office, January 1995, table 8, p.9.

Contact Bureau of Justice Statistics Clearinghouse, Box 6000, Rockville, MD 20850; (800) 732-3277. Drugs & Crime Data Center & Clearinghouse, 1600 Research Blvd., Rockville, MD 20850; (800) 666-3332.

Felony Convictions in State Courts: 1992

Number of felony convictions in state courts according to offense and type of conviction
(by jury trial or bench trial).

Offense	Jury Trial	Bench Trial	Trial Total	Guilty Plea	Total
Violent offenses	16,680	8,656	25,336	139,765	165,101
Murder	4,076	1,046	5,122	7,427	12,549
Rape	3,023	929	3,952	17,703	21,665
Robbery	3,860	2,225	6,085	45,794	51,879
Aggravated assault	4,409	3,053	7,462	51,507	58,969
Other violent offenses	1,312	1,404	2,716	17,333	20,049
Property offenses	7,473	8,681	16,154	281,340	297,494
Burglary	3,759	3,652	7,412	107,218	114,630
Larceny	2,668	4,049	6,717	112,283	119,000
Fraud	1,045	980	2,025	61,839	63,864
Drug offenses	8,567	12,663	21,230	259,001	280,231
Possession	1,839	8,039	9,878	99,548	109,426
Trafficking	6,728	4,624	11,352	159,453	170,805
Weapons offenses	1,205	1,126	2,331	24,091	26,422
Other offenses	3,668	4,249	7,917	116,465	124,382
All offenses	37,593	35,376	72,968	820,662	893,630

Comments Contrary to popular belief, neither murder nor violent crime generally accounts for most jury trials. Of all trial jury felony convictions in 1992, 44% (16,680 cases) were for violent crime; 56% (20,913 cases) were for nonviolent crime. The single felony category most frequently decided by juries was drug trafficking (6,728 cases, or 18% of all jury convictions), not murder (4,076 cases, or 11%).

Perhaps these drug trafficking cases occupy such a significant share of all trials by jury due to an increase in the use of the criminal justice system to deal with the drug problem.

Since the early 1980s, a special focus of many of the drug control policies implemented has been to increase the severity of punishment for drug trafficking. The goal of this approach is to interrupt the supply of illegal drugs. Although many people support this strategy, one drawback is the increase in public funds needed to handle the growing docket of drug offense cases.

Source U.S. Department of Justice. Office of Justice Programs. Bureau of Justice Statistics. *Felony Sentences in State Courts, 1992*. Washington, D.C.: U.S. Government Printing Office, January 1995, table 9, p.9.

Contact Bureau of Justice Statistics Clearinghouse, Box 6000, Rockville, MD 20850; (800) 732-3277. Drugs & Crime Data Center & Clearinghouse, 1600 Research Blvd., Rockville, MD 20850; (800) 666-3332.

Federal Drug Convictions: 1985–92

The number of defendants convicted in federal drug cases, according to type of drug offense.

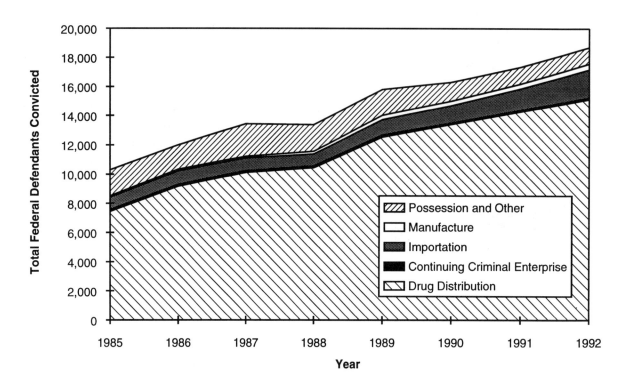

	1985	1986	1987	1988	1989	1990	1991	1992*	Percent Change 1985-92
Drug distribution	7,449	9,163	10,109	10,444	12,530	13,410	14,273	15,133	+103%
Continuing criminal enterprise	131	111	123	117	144	82	105	105	−20%
Importation	841	957	872	815	1,051	1,199	1,484	1,930	+129%
Manufacture	91	105	119	185	303	318	324	409	+349%
Possession and other	1,777	1,653	2,205	1,815	1,776	1,301	1,163	1,121	−37%
Total, all drug offenses	10,289	11,989	13,428	13,376	15,804	16,310	17,349	18,698	+82%

* Preliminary

Comments The composition of federal drug cases has changed since the mid-1980s. At that time, about 73% of all drug cases were for distribution (trafficking). Since then, however, the proportion of possession cases has declined, while the share of distribution cases increased to nearly 81% by 1992. From 1985 to 1992, the number of drug distribution convictions grew by 103%, while the number of possession cases shrank by 37%, as shown in the table.

Some of this change may be due to the added political emphasis given to the conviction of drug traffickers during these years. Convictions for manufacturing and importation increased by even greater shares, 349% and 129%, respectively. These three categories (manufacturing, importation, and distribution) focus primarily on the supply of illegal drugs. These supply-side activities have become the primary targets of the criminal justice system for dealing with the drug problem.

Source U.S. Department of Justice. Office of Justice Programs. Bureau of Justice Statistics. *Federal Drug Case Processing,* *1982–91, with Preliminary Data for 1992, a Federal Justice Statistics Report, NCJ-144392,* March 1994, table 7a, p. 5.

Contact Bureau of Justice Statistics Clearinghouse, Box 6000, Rockville, MD 20850; (800) 732-3277. Drugs & Crime Data Center & Clearinghouse, 1600 Research Blvd., Rockville, MD 20850; (800) 666-3332.

Federal Drug Control Spending: 1982–93

Federal drug control budgets (in $ millions) according to the type of control activity
during fiscal years 1982–93.

Year	International	Interdiction	Domestic Law Enforcement	Demand Reduction	Total*
1982	87.8	458.0	500.9	605.3	1,651.9
1983	83.9	473.5	692.1	685.2	1,934.7
1984	95.8	706.9	768.4	726.8	2,298.0
1985	109.2	807.3	969.2	793.9	2,679.6
1986	147.7	744.0	1,109.7	824.7	2,826.1
1987	220.9	1,350.5	1,791.9	1,423.4	4,786.7
1988	209.3	948.1	2,045.4	1,499.6	4,702.4
1989	304.0	1,440.7	2,814.8	2,032.8	6,592.3
1990	500.1	1,751.9	4,302.4	3,138.7	9,693.1
1991	639.6	2,027.9	4,489.0	3,684.9	10,841.4
1992	763.2	2,216.8	5,023.0	3,950.1	11,953.1
1993	767.9	2,219.6	5,490.2	4,250.5	12,728.7

* May not add due to rounding.

Comments The federal government has significantly increased its spending on drug control since the mid-1980s. Federal spending on drug control in 1989 was more than four times greater than spending in 1982, and 1993 expenditures were nearly double the 1989 amount. However, the level of spending for international efforts and for interdiction has grown very modestly.

Domestic law enforcement has grown significantly since the mid-1980s and now accounts for the largest portion of all spending. Demand reduction efforts have also quickly grown since the late 1980s to become the second largest category of spending.

By analyzing how the money was spent it is possible to understand which aspects of drug control are being emphasized. For instance, in the early 1980s interdiction represented a much larger portion of total spending than it does now. Domestic law enforcement now plays a much larger role in spending than it did in the early 1980s. In the early 1980s, demand reduction, domestic law enforcement, and interdiction were proportionately about the same in relation to total spending; by the early 1990s, the trend in spending clearly emphasized an agenda of domestic law enforcement first, followed by demand reduction, and then interdiction.

Source U.S. Department of Justice. Office of Justice Programs. Bureau of Justice Statistics. *Sourcebook of Criminal Justice Statistics—1992*. Washington, D.C.: U. S. Government Printing Office, [1993], table 1.16, pp. 19–21. Primary source: Executive Office of the President, Office of National Drug Control Policy, *National Drug Control Strategy: Budget Summary,* 1992, pp. 212–214.

Contact Bureau of Justice Statistics Clearinghouse, Box 6000, Rockville, MD 20850; (800) 732-3277. Drugs & Crime Data Center & Clearinghouse, 1600 Research Blvd., Rockville, MD 20850; (800) 666-3332. Executive Office of the President of the United States, Office of National Drug Control Policy, Washington, D.C. 20500; (202) 395-6700.

Federal Drug Control Spending by Function: 1995–96

Drug Function	1995/96 Estimate ($ millions)
Criminal Justice System	6,313.3
Drug Treatment	2,646.6
Education, Community Action, and the Workplace	1,847.6
International	309.9
Interdiction	1,293.3
Research	538.2
Intelligence	316.0
TOTAL	$13,264.9

Four-Way Split Functions	1995/96 Estimate ($ millions)
Demand Reduction	4,934.5
Domestic Law Enforcement	6,727.1
International	309.9
Interdiction	1,293.3
TOTAL	$13,264.9

Supply/Demand Split	1995/96 Estimate ($ millions)
Supply	8,330.3
Demand	4,934.5
TOTAL	$13,264.9

Comments These charts show how the federal government spent nearly $13.3 billion of its total budget toward drug control during fiscal year 1995. Each of the three charts accounts for the same $13,264.9 million but by different categories. Some federal agencies are exclusively drug control agencies (e.g., the Drug Enforcement Agency, the Office on National Drug Control Policy, and the Department of Justice Forfeiture Fund) but others vary widely in the proportion of their respective budgets used for drug control.

The first chart shows how the money was budgeted by drug function categories, which are composed of individual federal organizations focusing on some aspect of drug control. According to the first chart, about half of the budget went to the criminal justice system. A total of 48% was allocated to all the programs in various federal agencies that addressed drug control. The drug function categories are classifications that show how the federal expenditures immediately addressed the problem of drug control.

The second chart accounts for the same federal expenditures by their essential function in combating the drug problem. The categories included in this chart are broader than in the first, but give an insight into the strategic orientation of federal drug control policy (i.e., how the federal expenditures are actively addressing the problem rather than reacting to it).

The third chart shows the federal expenditures by the functions of supply and demand. The Anti-Drug Abuse Act of 1988 requires the Director of the Office of National Drug Control Policy to report on spending for programs dedicated to supply reduction and demand reduction activities. According to economics, all attempts at reducing the drug problem focus either on reducing the supply of illegal drugs to the market, or by influencing individuals to reduce their demand for illegal drugs.

Examples of supply-reduction tactics include drug and processing laboratory seizures, increased local and border policing. These methods increase the inconvenience or difficulty for an individual to acquire illegal drugs. Demand-reduction approaches include drug treatment and education programs, and any other method designed to influence an individual from seeking to use illicit drugs. Some methods, such as incarceration for drug offenders, may actually have a combined effect. When an offender who is a dealer is in prison, there will be a temporary interruption in the supply of drugs in his/her region of distribution. The imprisoned offender is also in a reasonably controlled environment and may be required to participate in a drug treatment program. The rehabilitation, coupled with the relative severity of a prison term, may persuade the offender that the perceived benefits of continued illegal drug use are not worth the inconvenience of losing his/her freedom.

Source Office of National Drug Control Policy. Executive Office of the President of the United States. *National Drug Control Strategy, Strengthening Communities'* *Response to Drugs and Crime, February 1995.* Washington, D.C.: U.S. Government Printing Office, [1995], table 9-1, p. 113.

Contact Executive Office of the President of the United States, Office of National Drug Control Policy, Washington, D.C. 20500; (202) 395-6700.

State and Local Drug Control Spending: 1991

Drug control spending (in $ millions) at the state and local levels,
according to type of control activity for fiscal year 1991.

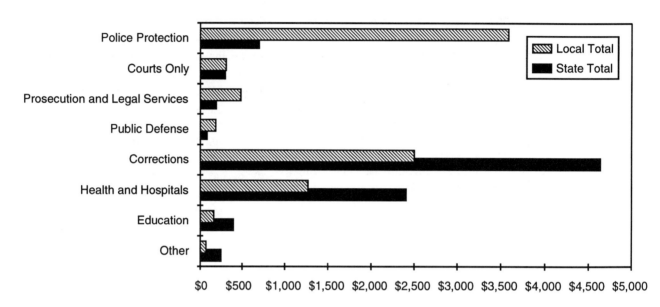

**Drug Control Expenditure
(millions of dollars)**

	State			Local			
	Direct	Inter-governmental	State Total	Direct	Inter-governmental	Local Total	All State and Local
Police protection	637	57	695	3,585	1	3,586	4,223
Courts only	228	74	303	311	1	313	540
Prosecution and legal services	168	27	195	482	1	483	649
Public defense	73	6	80	187	—	187	260
Corrections	4,342	296	4,638	2.486	14	2,500	6,827
Health & hospitals	1,611	794	2,405	1,173	94	1,268	2,784
Education	340	60	399	163	—	163	503
Other	53	198	251	68	—	68	120
TOTAL	$7,451	$1,513	$8,965	$8,455	$112	$8,567	$15,907

Comments

Public spending for controlling the illicit drug trade differs between the federal, state, and local levels by function.

According to the table shown here, during fiscal year 1991 state governments spent a greater amount of public funds on drug control measures than did local governments (about $400 million more). Direct payments are expenditures taken from the revenue of the state or local government's own tax base. Intergovernmental expenditures consist of payments from one government to another; such expenditures eventually show up as direct expenditures of the receiving government.

Although the expenditures by state and local governments are similar in amount, the proportions of the expenditures by function differ significantly between the two. These expenditures vary because state and local governments have different priorities and responsibilities. For example, the largest expenditure category for state governments was corrections, which accounted for over 51% of total expenditures by all state governments for drug control that year. On the other hand, expenditures for corrections by local governments only amounted to 29% of total local expenditures, but spending for police protection accounted for nearly 42%.

Source

Office of National Drug Control Policy. Executive Office of the President of the United States. *National Drug Control Strategy, Strengthening Communities' Response to Drugs and Crime, February 1995.* Washington, D.C.: U.S. Government Printing Office, [1995], p. 138. Primary source: Office of National Drug Control Policy.

Contact

Executive Office of the President of the United States, Office of National Drug Control Policy, Washington, D.C., 20500; (202) 395-6700.

Drug Enforcement by Local and State Law Enforcement Agencies: 1990

Percentage of sheriffs' and local and state police departments with primary responsibility for enforcement of narcotics laws, according to the type of department and number of population served.

Type of Agency and Population Served	Number	Percent with Primary Narcotics Enforcement
Sheriffs'	**3,093**	**81%**
1,000,000 or more	27	74%
500,000 to 999,999	62	56%
250,000 to 499,999	92	60%
100,000 to 249,999	270	67%
50,000 to 99,999	374	80%
Under 50,000	2,268	84%
Local police	**12,228**	**76%**
1,000,000 or more	14	100%
500,000 to 999,999	29	97%
250,000 to 499,999	42	100%
100,000 to 249,999	137	99%
50,000 to 99,999	344	96%
Under 50,000	11,722	75%
State police	**49**	**34%**
TOTAL	**15,430**	**77%**

Comments

The burden of drug enforcement falls heavily on local law enforcement agencies, particularly sheriffs' departments, which typically serve suburban and rural populations. Local police forces, except in the smallest municipalities, make up a significant segment of the nation's primary narcotics enforcement agencies. Overall, more than 75% of all state and local law enforcement agencies have the primary responsibility of narcotics enforcement.

Many law enforcement agencies may have jurisdiction over one incident or network. Typically, one agency will take the lead in a drug case, depending on the agency's capabilities, policies, and procedures. For example, the trial of an arrestee in a U.S. district court may be the result of a joint federal/local investigation into a drug distribution ring. The arrestee is being held in federal court because the law enforcement agencies involved believe the case has a better chance for conviction under the rules of evidence and procedure in that court.

Source

U.S. Department of Justice. Office of Justice Programs. Bureau of Justice Statistics. *Drugs, Crime, and the Justice System, A National Report from the Bureau of Justice Statistics, December 1992, NCJ-133652.* Washington, D.C.: U.S. Government Printing Office, [1992], p. 142. Primary source: Bureau of Justice Statistics, *Drug Enforcement by Police and Sheriffs' Departments, 1990,* Special Report, May 1992, table 1.

Contact

Bureau of Justice Statistics Clearinghouse, Box 6000, Rockville, MD 20850; (800) 732-3277. Drugs & Crime Data Center & Clearinghouse, 1600 Research Blvd., Rockville, MD 20850; (800) 666-3332.

Multiagency Drug Enforcement Task Force Participants: 1990

Types of local and state law enforcement agencies participating in multiagency drug enforcement task forces, by percent of agencies and numbers of officers assigned.

Type of Agency and Population Served	Percent of Agencies Participating	Total Number of Full-Time Officers Assigned	Average Number of Full-Time Officers Assigned
Sheriffs'	**68%**	**3,514**	**2**
1,000,000 or more	95%	190	10
500,000 to 999,999	97%	230	7
250,000 to 499,999	91%	375	8
100,000 to 249,999	86%	618	4
50,000 to 99,999	72%	564	3
25,000 to 49,999	80%	533	1
10,000 to 24,999	66%	698	1
Under 10,000	49%	306	1
Local police	**51%**	**6,109**	**1**
1,000,000 or more	93%	382	29
500,000 to 999,999	100%	199	7
250,000 to 499,999	87%	262	7
100,000 to 249,999	86%	496	4
50,000 to 99,999	81%	576	2
25,000 to 49,999	82%	837	2
10,000 to 24,999	65%	1,162	1
2,500 to 9,999	55%	1,576	1
Under 2,500	28%	618	1
State police	**91%**	**986**	**29**

Comments Law enforcement agencies are compelled to join together in their efforts to combat the drug trafficking problem. Drug traffickers operate across local, state, and even federal boundaries. Such coordination is either vertical, involving many jurisdictions, or horizontal, involving agencies at various levels of government.

According to these statistics, in 1990 there were over 10,000 full-time local and state law enforcement officers assigned to multiagency drug task forces. Cases that require a multiagency approach at the federal level are handled by the Organized Crime Drug Enforcement Task Force (OCDETF). In 1988, cocaine was involved in 80% of the investigations conducted by the OCDETF; marijuana, 45%; heroin, 24%; methamphetamine, 11%; hashish, 5%; methaqualone, 5%; and PCP, 3%.

Many local and state agencies also participate in the 44 formal and 12 provisional task forces funded by the DEA. According to the Criminal Justice Statistics Association, more than 700 multijurisdictional drug control task forces operate with funding provided by the Anti-Drug Abuse Acts of 1986 and 1988.

Source U.S. Department of Justice. Office of Justice Programs. Bureau of Justice Statistics. *Drugs, Crime, and the Justice System, A National Report from the Bureau of Justice Statistics, December 1992, NCJ-133652.* Washington, D.C.: U.S. Government Printing Office, [1992], p. 149. Primary source: Bureau of Justice Statistics, *Drug Enforcement by Police and Sheriffs' Departments, 1990*, Special Report, May 1992, table 4.

Contact Bureau of Justice Statistics Clearinghouse, Box 6000, Rockville, MD 20850; (800) 732-3277. Drugs & Crime Data Center & Clearinghouse, 1600 Research Blvd., Rockville, MD 20850; (800) 666-3332.

Federal Seizures of Marijuana, Cocaine, and Heroin: 1989–93

The prevalence of federal seizures by weight (in kilograms) of marijuana (cannabis), cocaine, and heroin, with accommodations for the weight/potency differences among these narcotics.

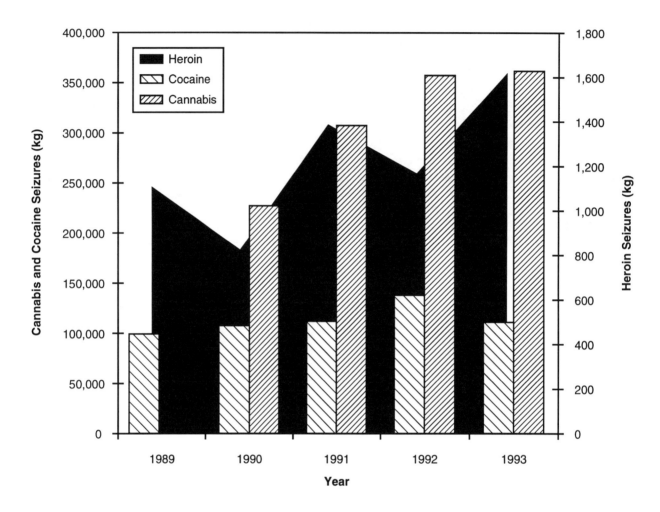

Year	Cannabis (kg)	Cocaine (kg)	Heroin (kg)
1989	—	99,200	1,095.2
1990	226,984	107,300	815.0
1991	307,212	111,700	1374.4
1992	357,159	137,800	1,157.2
1993	361,624	110,700	1,600.9

Comments These graphs indicate the prevalence of federal seizures of cannabis (marijuana), cocaine, and heroin in recent years. There are two different graphs to accommodate for the weight differences for the seizures of heroin. If heroin were included on the same graph as cannabis and cocaine, it would appear as a nearly flat line along the bottom of the graph because of the scale used to measure the kilograms seized for the other two drugs. According to the first graph, cannabis seizures have risen since 1990, while cocaine seizures by weight have remained more stable. What these two lines fail to address, however, is the fact that cocaine is a much more potent drug than cannabis. One kilogram of cocaine seized will have a greater economic impact on drug trafficking than will one kilogram of cannabis. Heroin seizures, however, seem to be on the rise but fluctuate from year to year, according to the years analyzed by these statistics.

Source Federal-wide Drug Seizure System, Drug Enforcement Administration as cited by the Executive Office of the President of the United States, *National Drug Control Strategy*, p. 145.

Contact Drug Enforcement Administration, 600-700 Army Navy Dr., Arlington, VA 22202. Public Affairs: (202)307-7977. Drugs & Crime Data Center & Clearinghouse, 1600 Research Blvd., Rockville, MD 20850: (800) 666-3332.

Land and Marine Seizures of Marijuana and Cocaine: 1976–92

Number of pounds of marijuana and cocaine seized by U.S. Customs (land border smuggling)
and the U.S. Coast Guard (smuggling at sea), for fiscal years 1976–92.

Year	Marijuana Seizures		Cocaine Seizures	
	U.S. Customs Service	U.S. Coast Guard	U.S. Customs Service	U.S. Coast Guard
1976	759,359.9	183,168	1,029.6	62.00
1977	1,652,772.7	1,032,609	952.1	0.00
1978	4,616,883.7	3,321,035	1,418.7	0.00
1979	3,583,555.5	2,682,586	1,438.1	0.00
1980	2,361,141.5	2,494,774	4,742.9	0.00
1981	5,109,792.5	2,643,043	3,741.1	40.00
1982	3,958,870.9	3,525,775	11,149.5	9.36
1983	2,732,974.5	2,448,940	19,601.5	46.20
1984	3,274,927.2	2,505,357	27,525.8	1,966.92
1985	2,389,704.1	2,142,133	50,506.4	6,546.82
1986	2,211,068.1	1,523,070	52,520.9	10,333.66
1987	1,701,149.6	1,212,963	87,898.3	14,723.42
1988	969,966.7	448,894	137,408.4	12,825.56
1989	645,858.2	224,606	129,493.2	32,896.00
1990	222,313.8	62,279	164,727.0	15,152.68
1991	287,519.5	22,145	169,586.1	29,033.02
1992	462,831.0	44,585	244,597.2	14,449.96

Comments

Interdiction is a method used to keep illegal drugs from being entered into the U.S. from abroad by intercepting and seizing the contraband. The U.S. Customs Service is responsible for interdicting land border smuggling. The U.S. Coast Guard is in charge of preventing marine drug smuggling on the high seas. These two federal agencies share responsibility for interdicting smuggling in coastal waters and for stopping air smuggling. The Department of Defense is the lead agency in the detection and monitoring of aerial and maritime transit of illegal drugs into the U.S., but the military is prohibited from making arrests. Other federal agencies involved in interdiction include the Drug Enforcement Administration, the Immigration and Naturalization Service's Border Patrol, and the Federal Aviation Administration.

Cargo, vessels, and passengers entering the U.S. at ports are inspected by the U.S. Customs Service. The use of dogs trained to smell and find illegal drugs hidden in vehicles and cargo is one tactic used by the U.S. Customs Service, and has led to more than 75,000 narcotics seizures since 1970. Air interdiction, however, is more difficult because of the enormous volume of legitimate commercial and private air traffic. Also, once they are detected, air smugglers often ignore directions to land, jettison their illegal cargo, and flee. Marine interdiction attempts to stop ships from delivering their cargo of illegal drugs to dropoff points just outside the U.S. The U.S. Coast Guard has cooperative programs with several foreign law enforcement agencies to allow the pursuit of smugglers into foreign waters.

This chart illustrates seizures of marijuana and cocaine—the two drugs most often intercepted through the interdiction efforts of the U.S. Customs Service and the U.S. Coast Guard. According to these statistics, the amount of marijuana seized in recent years has fallen significantly, while the amount of cocaine seized by U.S. Customs has escalated. The drop in marijuana seizures could mean that fewer people are smuggling that particular drug into the U.S., or that fewer smugglers are being detected through interdiction, or that the smugglers have adopted another means to get marijuana into the country. The disparity in the trend of cocaine seizures between the two agencies could mean that more people are smuggling cocaine indirectly through port traffic than directly over the high seas, or that the situations and/or techniques of interdiction utilized by the U.S. Customs Service lend themselves to greater success than those of the U.S. Coast Guard. By analyzing these trends in seizures, it is possible to make a general assumption that since 1980, the total annual weight for seizures has decreased for marijuana but increased for cocaine. It is not possible, however, to explain why these trends exist with the information given here.

Source

U.S. Department of Justice. Office of Justice Programs. Bureau of Justice Statistics. *Drugs, Crime, and the Justice System, A National Report from the Bureau of Justice Statistics, December 1992, NCJ-133652.* Washington, D.C.: U.S. Government Printing Office, [1992], pp. 146–147. U.S. Department of Justice. Office of Justice Programs. Bureau of Justice Statistics. *Sourcebook of Criminal Justice Statistics—1992,* Washington, D.C.: U.S. Government Printing Office, [1993], pp. 466–7, 470–1.

Contact

U.S. Department of the Treasury, U.S. Customs Service, 1301 Constitution Ave. NW, Washington, DC 20229, Public Affairs: (202) 566-8195. U.S. Department of Transportation, U.S. Coast Guard 2100 Second St. SW, Washington, DC 20593. Maritime Law Enforcement: (202)267-1890.

Seizures of Illegal Drug Laboratories: 1975–91

Secret drug laboratories seized by the Drug Enforcement Administration (DEA) in fiscal years 1975–91 according to the major type of drug manufactured.

Year	PCP	Amphetamine	Methamphetamine	Other	TOTAL
1975	15	2	11	4	32
1976	30	11	36	20	97
1977	66	10	46	26	148
1978	79	12	69	20	180
1979	53	10	137	35	235
1980	49	20	126	39	234
1981	35	14	87	46	182
1982	47	18	132	27	224
1983	39	25	119	43	226
1984	13	19	121	44	197
1985	23	67	257	72	419
1986	8	66	372	63	509
1987	13	68	561	40	682
1988	20	82	667	41	810
1989	13	10	683	55	852
1990	10	54	449	36	549
1991	5	25	327	30	387

Comments

Secret laboratories are often used by drug traffickers to process and refine illicit drugs, such as methamphetamine, amphetamine, PCP, methaqualone, and LSD. This table illustrates the number of such secret laboratories seized by the DEA from 1975 to 1990.

According to the table, these seizures escalated rapidly after 1984 and peaked in 1989. However, since the table only reports seized laboratories, it is not possible to know exactly how many laboratories remained secret in any particular year. In 1990, some 82% of these seized laboratories produced methamphetamine; 10% produced amphetamine; and 3% produced P2P—a precursor to methamphetamine.

Most of the 549 laboratories seized in 1990 were in the western (55%) or south central states (30%). Secret labs are set up by drug organizations in rural as well as urban areas. Some labs are even portable and are moved after producing several batches in one location. These labs are not only a threat to law enforcement, but are often a safety hazard to the community—about 20% of all secret laboratories discovered are noticed through, or result in, a fire or explosion. Clandestine laboratories also use many chemicals that are reactive, explosive, flammable, corrosive, or toxic. This poses an environmental hazard when chemicals and by-products of the manufacturing process are disposed of indiscriminately to avoid detection.

Source

U.S. Department of Justice. Office of Justice Programs. Bureau of Justice Statistics. *Drugs, Crime, and the Justice System, A National Report from the Bureau of Justice Statistics, December 1992, NCJ-133652.* Washington, D.C.: U.S. Government Printing Office, [1992], p. 151. Primary source: Drug Enforcement Administration, as presented in Bureau of Justice Statistics, *Sourcebook of Criminal Justice Statistics, 1990, NCJ-130580,* p. 467. U.S. Department of Justice. Office of Justice Programs. Bureau of Justice Statistics. *Sourcebook of Criminal Justice Statistics—1992.* Washington, D.C.: U. S. Government Printing Office, [1993], table 4.32, p. 469. Primary source: Comptroller General of the United States, *Report to Congress: Stronger Crackdown Needed on Clandestine Laboratories Manufacturing Dangerous Drugs,* 1981, p. 37; also, data provided by U.S. Department of Justice, Drug Enforcement Administration.

Contact

Drug Enforcement Administration, 600-700 Army Navy Dr., Arlington, VA 22202. Public Affairs: (202)307-7977. Drugs & Crime Data Center & Clearinghouse, 1600 Research Blvd., Rockville, MD 20850; (800) 666-3332.

International Drug Seizures: 1989–93

Estimated international seizures of particular drugs, measured in metric tons.
Also, average percent each drug contributes to overall seizures.

Average Percent of International Drug Seizures

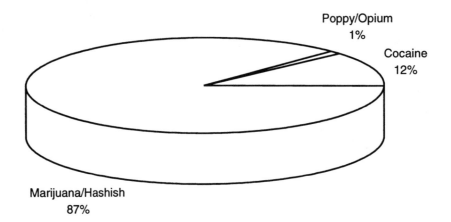

	1989	1990	1991	1992	1993
Poppy/Opium	30	26	26	24	41
Cocaine	250	275	345	285	265
Marijuana/Hashish	1,496	2,261	1,603	2,303	2,886

Comments One way to reduce the supply of drugs is to increase the difficulty for drug traffickers to transport drugs into the U.S. The trends in international drug seizures between 1989 and 1993, as shown in the accompanying table, have shown an increase in poppy/opium and marijuana/hashish seizures, but a drop in cocaine seizures. Currently, about one-third of the potential worldwide supply of cocaine is eventually seized, with the U.S. accounting for about one-third to one-half of these seizures.

A decline in international seizures for a particular drug could mean one or more of the following: a drop in overall production (less is seized because less is produced); more effective smuggling methods; less effective interdiction methods by law enforcement agencies, a shift in transportation methods by smugglers; or increased corruption of law enforcement personnel, resulting in collaboration with smugglers.

Source Office of National Drug Control Policy. Executive Office of the President of the United States. *National Drug Control Strategy, Strengthening Communities' Response to Drugs and Crime, February 1995.* Washington, D.C.: U.S. Government Printing Office, [1995], p. 48. Primary source: Bureau of International Narcotics Matters, 1994, United Nations International Drug Control Programme, 1994, and Office of National Drug Control Policy intelligence estimates.

Contact Executive Office of the President of the United States, Office of National Drug Control Policy, Washington, D.C. 20500; (202) 395-6700.

Destruction of Cannabis Plants in the States: 1982–90

Efforts of the DEA (Drug Enforcement Administration) to destroy cannabis (marijuana) plants in various states, by number of plants destroyed each year.

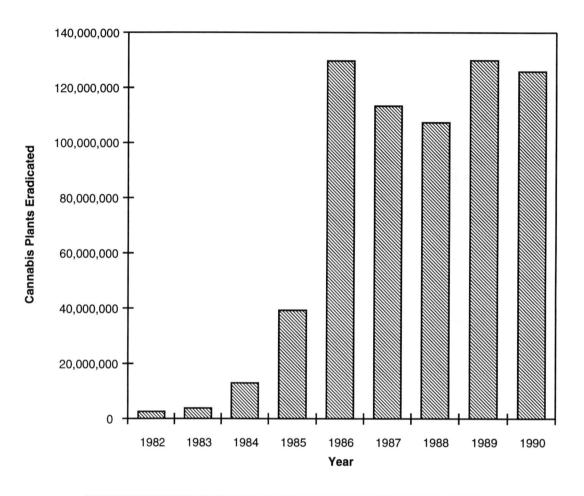

Year	Number of States	Plants Eradicated
1982	25	2,590,388
1983	40	3,793,943
1984	50	12,981,210
1985	50	39,231,479
1986	49	129,686,033
1987	46	113,274,824
1988	47	107,276,308
1989	49	129,924,695
1990	50	125,876,752

Comments In 1979, the Drug Enforcement Administration (DEA) began the Domestic Cannabis Eradication/Suppression Program. This program gives financial and technical assistance, training, and equipment to state and local agencies. In 1990, all fifty states participated in the program. Through this data table, it is possible to get a general idea of the program's accomplishments. It is difficult to compare one year's eradications with another's, since the number of states engaged in the program varied from year to year.

Through this program, the DEA cooperates with the U.S. Forest Service, the Bureau of Land Management, the Fish and Wildlife Service, the National Park Service, the Bureau of Indian Affairs, and the Department of Defense.

The destruction of cannabis plants is very labor intensive and often involves local National Guard personnel. Including the efforts of the DEA, state, and local enforcement agencies, over 29,000 cannabis plots and 7.3 million cultivated plants were destroyed in 1990. Of the total number of plants removed, about 2 million were sinsemilla (young female plants with the highest THC content). About 70% of the sinsemilla annihilated was located in Missouri, Hawaii, and Tennessee. Officials also eradicated over 118 million ditchweed plants (a low potency cannabis that grows wild in many parts of the U.S.), mostly in Indiana and Nebraska.

Source U.S. Department of Justice. Office of Justice Programs. Bureau of Justice Statistics. *Drugs, Crime, and the Justice System, A National Report from the Bureau of Justice Statistics, December 1992, NCJ-* *133652.* Washington, D.C.: U.S. Government Printing Office, [1992], p.150. Primary source: Drug Enforcement Administration, 1990 Domestic Cannabis Eradication/Suppression Program, 1991, p. 10.

Contact Drug Enforcement Administration, 600-700 Army Navy Dr., Arlington, VA 22202. Public Affairs: (202) 307-7977. National Clearinghouse for Drug and Alcohol Information: (800) 729-6686.

Cannabis Eradication Efforts: 1990

Results of the combined federal, state, and local DEA cannabis eradication programs,
ranked by number of plants seized and destroyed in each state.

Rank	State	Cultivated Plants	Plots Eradicated	Indoor Grow Sites Seized
1	Missouri	1,141,687	609	30
2	Oklahoma	1,013,036	605	9
3	Nebraska	760,523	27	8
4	Hawaii	752,937	2,068	10
5	Kentucky	616,289	3,189	24
6	Tennessee	542,580	2,796	177
7	Michigan	311,206	786	51
8	Illinois	288,167	304	43
9	California	199,105	2,084	263
10	Alabama	192,918	1,831	4
11	Minnesota	187,349	315	16
12	Indiana	187,107	1,965	8
13	North Carolina	145,916	2,511	19
14	Arkansas	125,420	1,541	22
15	Wisconsin	107,940	376	58
16	Georgia	97,233	1,378	2
17	Florida	92,901	1,148	45
18	Texas	69,865	523	28
19	Oregon	59,785	1,057	281
20	Mississippi	53,066	380	0
21	Pennsylvania	51,673	199	4
22	Louisiana	44,596	377	31
23	Ohio	43,437	485	63
24	Virginia	33,660	619	39
25	Washington	30,801	280	178
26	West Virginia	25,350	220	3
27	Arizona	24,760	17	6
28	South Carolina	23,636	238	5
29	Kansas	18,289	290	27
30	Maine	13,729	254	16
31	Iowa	12,027	102	3
32	South Dakota	10,774	32	1
33	Alaska	8,637	41	41
34	Vermont	5,585	77	4
35	New Mexico	4,447	25	2
36	New York	4,283	100	1
37	Colorado	3,846	30	6

[Continued]

Cannabis Eradication Efforts: 1990

[Continued]

Rank	State	Cultivated Plants	Plots Eradicated	Indoor Grow Sites Seized
38	Montana	3,730	26	25
39	Massachusetts	3,444	72	22
40	Idaho	3,194	38	27
41	Maryland	2,886	316	8
42	New Hampshire	2,542	61	31
43	Nevada	2,200	15	6
44	North Dakota	1,761	10	5
45	Utah	1,582	13	4
46	Wyoming	1,291	8	7
47	New Jersey	526	11	1
48	Rhode Island	500	16	5
49	Connecticut	326	3	0
50	Delaware	227	1	0

Comments The Domestic Cannabis Eradication/Suppression Program, operated by the Drug Enforcement Administration (DEA), is a cooperative effort between federal, state, and local law enforcement agencies to reduce the quantity of marijuana grown in the U.S. In 1990, every state participated in this program. The accompanying table shows each state ranked by the number of plants seized and destroyed through the efforts of this program.

Some smaller states like Hawaii accounted for a considerable number of the eradicated plants, while larger states like Montana accounted for a small proportion of the national total. Some of this difference can explained by the more favorable growing climate in Hawaii relative to Montana. Some states may also have more fertile remote growing regions than others, or better access to distribution networks.

The number of indoor operations seized has been on the rise in recent years, increasing from 951 operations in 1985 to 1,669 in 1990. The DEA has developed a Special Enforcement Operation, "Operation Green Merchant." It targets suppliers of cannabis seeds, growing equipment, cultivation information, and the growers. In 1989, Operation Green Merchant resulted in 441 arrests, the dismantling of 356 operations, and seizure of 48,744 sinsemilla plants and almost 1 ton of processed marijuana.

Source U.S. Department of Justice. Office of Justice Programs. Bureau of Justice Statistics. *Drugs, Crime, and the Justice System, A National Report from the Bureau of Justice Statistics, December 1992, NCJ-133652.* Washington, D.C.: U.S. Government Printing Office, [1992], p. 150. Primary source: Drug Enforcement Administration, 1990 Domestic Cannabis Eradication/Suppression Program, 1991, pp. 6-9.

Contact Drug Enforcement Administration, 600-700 Army Navy Dr., Arlington, VA 22202. Public Affairs: (202) 307-7977. National Clearinghouse for Alcohol and Drug Information: (800) 729-6686.

State and Local Narcotics Enforcement: 1990

Percentage of state and local law enforcement agencies with primary drug enforcement responsibilities that seized illegal drugs, listed by type of agency, population served, and drug type seized.

Type of Agency and Population Served	Pow-dered Cocaine	Crack Cocaine	Heroin	Mari-juana	LSD	PCP	Stimu-lants	Depress-ants	Designer Drugs
Sheriffs'	**71%**	**44%**	**18%**	**94%**	**33%**	**13%**	**60%**	**35%**	**15%**
250,000 or more	94	88	80	99	78	44	90	67	36
100,000 to 249,999	97	79	48	95	66	32	75	57	28
25,000 to 99,999	86	53	21	96	46	20	72	52	21
Under 25,000	58	31	7	92	17	5	49	20	7
Local police	**63%**	**42%**	**19%**	**86%**	**25%**	**10%**	**44%**	**28%**	**10%**
250,000 or more	100	99	96	98	92	59	96	75	57
100,000 to 249,999	97	92	85	99	76	43	88	62	43
25,000 to 99,999	95	76	56	95	54	26	77	51	23
Under 25,000	58	37	12	85	19	7	39	24	7
State police	**100%**	**91%**	**91%**	**100%**	**88%**	**74%**	**94%**	**88%**	**53%**

Comments   Most state and local agencies, having the principal responsibility for narcotics enforcement, made seizures of illegal drugs in 1990. That year, 49 state police agencies reported seizing powdered cocaine and marijuana. Marijuana was the most common drug seized by both local police and sheriffs' departments. A greater proportion of all sheriffs' departments made seizures of marijuana than local police departments. Powdered cocaine, however, was seized by every local police department in the nation that serves a population of more than 250,000 inhabitants.

This table shows how common it was in 1990 for a particular type of law enforcement agency to make a seizure of a specific type of illegal drug. Of the three types of agencies listed here, state police agencies generally had the largest geographical domain to cover, followed by sheriffs' departments, and local police forces.

Source   U.S. Department of Justice. Office of Justice Programs. Bureau of Justice Statistics. *Drugs, Crime, and the Justice System, A National Report from the Bureau of Justice Statistics, December 1992, NCJ-133652*. Washington, D.C.: U.S. Government Printing Office, [1992], p. 152. Primary source: Bureau of Justice Statistics, *Drug Enforcement by Police and Sheriffs' Departments, 1990*, Special Report, May 1992.

Contact   Bureau of Justice Statistics Clearinghouse, Box 6000, Rockville, MD 20850; (800) 732-3277. Drugs & Crime Data Center & Clearinghouse, 1600 Research Blvd., Rockville, MD 20850; (800) 666-3332.

Asset Seizure by the DEA: 1992

Types and values of assets seized by the Drug Enforcement Administration's efforts to stop illegal drug trade in fiscal year 1992.

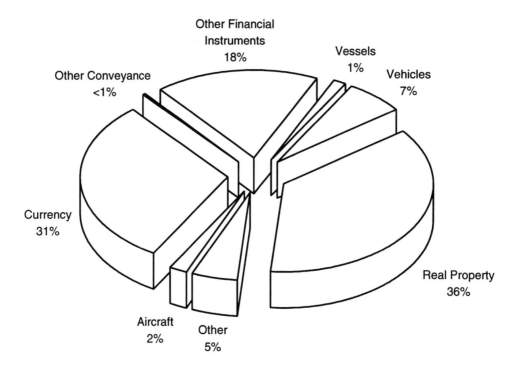

Asset Seizure by the DEA, 1992
(percent)

Type of Asset	Value	Number of Seizures
Real property	320,631,938	1,712
Vehicles	57,065,862	5,948
Aircraft	15,828,500	53
Vessels	12,399,302	228
Other conveyances	2,146,124	278
Other	44,162,856	2,564
Currency	267,820,145	8,344
Other financial instruments	154,834,673	741
TOTAL	$874,889,400	19,868

Comments Drug traffickers are in the business primarily to make money. Asset forfeiture and money laundering laws are aimed at stripping away assets and profits from those who earn money from the illicit drug trade. Asset forfeiture laws attempt to permanently curtail the financial ability of criminal organizations to maintain their illegal operations. Most forfeiture laws originally targeted the seizure of contraband, or modes of transporting or distributing such materials.

Common provisions permit the seizure of airplanes, boats, cars, the materials and equipment used in manufacturing, and drug paraphernalia. Since the 1970s, the types of property that may be forfeited have been expanded to include assets derived from criminal activity such as cash, securities, negotiable instruments, real property (including houses and other real estate), and proceeds gained directly or indirectly through violations of drug or money laundering laws. Seized property purchased with illegal proceeds has also included jewelry, businesses, art objects, livestock, and exotic animals.

Asset seizures dramatically increased during the 1980s. By 1990, about two-thirds of the DEA's seizures were the result of cocaine investigations and about one-fifth resulted from cannabis investigations. Despite the laundering efforts of drug traffickers, drug money is subject to forfeiture even if it is mixed in with legitimate assets. Some people consider law enforcement's focus on drug proceeds and assets a reactive or defensive strategy, utilized after the inability to control illegal drugs at the earlier stages of cultivation, marketing, manufacturing, and smuggling.

Source U.S. Department of Justice. Office of Justice Programs. Bureau of Justice Statistics. *Sourcebook of Criminal Justice Statistics—1992*. Washington, D.C.: U. S. Government Printing Office, [1993], table 4.43, p.

469. Primary source: Data provided by the U.S. Department of Justice, Drug Enforcement Administration, Computerized Asset Program.

Contact Drug Enforcement Administration, 600-700 Army Navy Dr., Arlington, VA 22202. Public Affairs: (202) 307-7977.

National Clearinghouse for Drug and Alcohol Information: (800) 729-6686.

Federal Asset Forfeiture Funds: 1986–90

Asset forfeiture funds from seizures from criminal organizations (in $ millions).

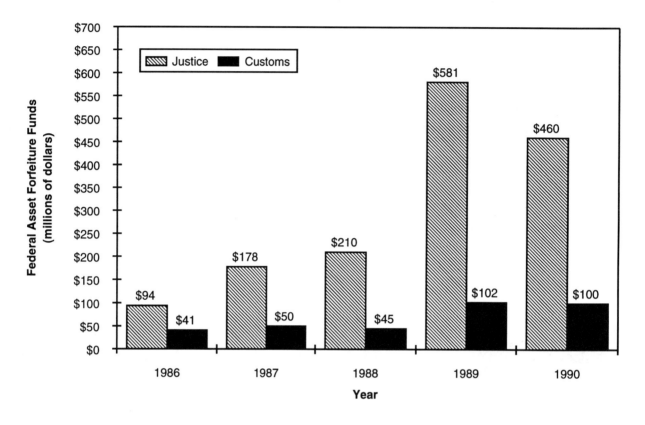

Year	Justice	Customs
1986	$94	$41
1987	$178	$50
1988	$210	$45
1989	$581*	$102
1990	$460	$100

* Includes $222 million from the Drexel Burnham securities fraud case.

The 1984 Comprehensive Drug Abuse and Prevention Act established the Department of Justice Asset Forfeiture Fund and the Customs Forfeiture Fund for customs law forfeitures. Agencies that participate include the Drug Enforcement Administration (DEA), the FBI, the U.S. Marshals Service, the Immigration and Naturalization Service, as well as the U.S. Postal Inspection Service, the Internal Revenue Service, and the Bureau of Alcohol, Tobacco, and Firearms.

Within the Department of Justice, the U.S. Marshals Service is responsible for managing and liquidating property, often through public sales and auctions. Since the 1980s, both these forfeiture funds have grown. In 1990, the largest dispersal from the Department of Justice Asset Forfeiture Fund went to other governments as part of an international asset-sharing program, fostered by improved cooperation by foreign governments with U.S. officials in money-laundering cases. Significant funds are also transferred to various federal law enforcement agencies. Funds transferred to the Office of National Drug Control Policy are used to support the construction of federal prisons.

Source U.S. Department of Justice. Office of Justice Programs. Bureau of Justice Statistics. *Drugs, Crime, and the Justice System, A National Report from the Bureau of Justice Statistics, December 1992, NCJ-133652*. Washington, D.C.: U.S. Government Printing Office, [1992], p. 157. Primary source: Office of National Drug Control Policy and the U.S. Marshals Service.

Contact Executive Office of the President of the United States, Office of National Drug Control Policy, Washington, D.C. 20500; (202) 395-6700.

Monthly Drug-Related Personal Income

Income reported by drug users from legal and illegal sources.

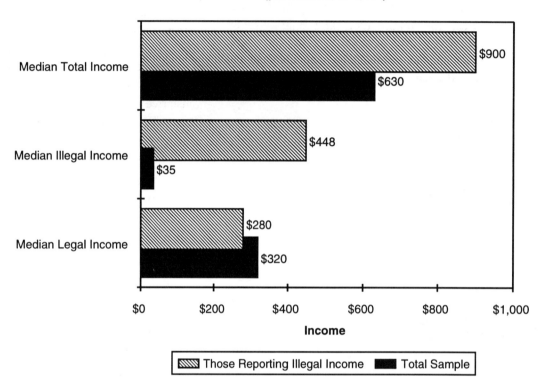

**Median Income Amounts
(past month, N=1,154)**

Legal Sources (of those with any legal income)	
Public assistance	47%
Paid job, salary, self-employment	46%
Family, friends	38%
Social Security, disability	13%
Unemployment	2%
Illegal Sources (of those with any illegal income)	
Drug-related (median amount $450)	42%
Property crime (median amount $450)	30%
Commercial sex (median amount $300)	42%
Violent crimes	2%

Comments

The National Institute on Drug Abuse conducted a study on the extent of illegal economic activity by drug users, as indicated by the accompanying chart. According to this study, drug users who are not in treatment have a high incidence of criminal activity. About one-half of the respondents in the study reported having only legal income. The other half also had illegal income sources, which included drug-related, property, and commercial sex crimes. The majority of drug users had some sort of legal income; only 10% derived their income solely through illegal means.

Legal income was most commonly obtained from public assistance, followed by paid labor and remittances from family and friends. For individuals reporting illegal income, the average monthly legitimate income only accounted for about one-third of average total monthly income. Such information indicates that chronic illicit drug abusers often become experienced in other illegal behaviors as well.

Source

Office of National Drug Control Policy. Executive Office of the President of the United States. *National Drug Control Strategy, Strengthening Communities' Response to Drugs and Crime, February 1995.* Washington, D.C.: U.S. Government Printing Office, [1995], pp. 34–35. Primary source: National Institute on Drug Abuse, *Drug Procurement Practices of the Out-of-Treatment Chronic Abuser*, 1994.

Contact

Executive Office of the President of the United States, Office of National Drug Control Policy, Washington, D.C. 20500; (202) 395-6700.

Total U.S. Expenditures on Illicit Drugs: 1988–93

Estimated billions of dollars spent on selected illegal drugs, showing trends in use.

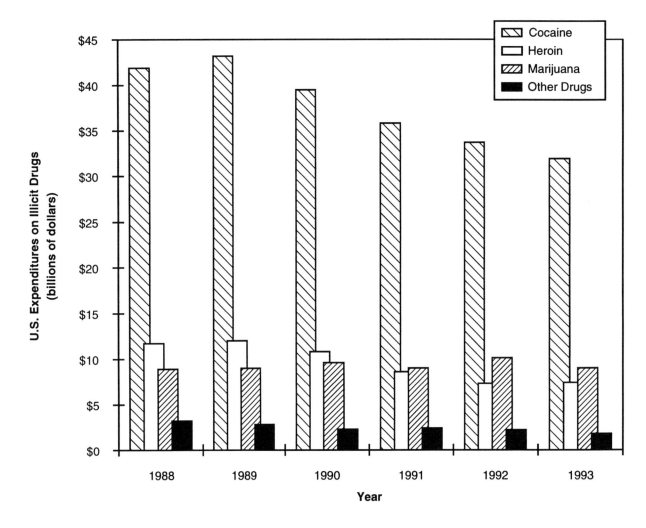

	1988	1989	1990	1991	1992	1993
Cocaine	41.9	43.2	39.5	35.8	33.7	31.9
Heroin	11.7	12.0	10.8	8.6	7.3	7.4
Marijuana	8.9	9.0	9.6	9.0	10.1	9.0
Other drugs	3.2	2.8	2.3	2.4	2.2	1.8
TOTAL	$65.7	$66.9	$62.2	$55.9	$53.3	$50.1

Comments This chart gives an overall estimate of the amount of money users spent on illegal drugs during the years specified. Since 1989, the amount has decreased. This does not necessarily mean that drug use has decreased. If, for instance, the price of drugs fell after 1989, the same amount or even more could be consumed with fewer dollars. But according to other sources, the smaller expenditure on illicit drugs is related to a decreased demand reflecting decreased use. Still, in 1993 Americans spent over $50 billion on illegal drugs.

Although the total amount spent for illegal drugs has decreased since 1989, the proportions spent for specific drugs have remained relatively constant.

For instance, cocaine varied between 63-65% of all illegal drug expenditures; other illicit drugs (amphetamines, barbiturates, methaqualone, etc.), represented the smallest proportion at 4–5%. The proportions of expenditures in both these categories—compared to all the money spent for illegal drugs—are more stable than are the expenditures for heroin or marijuana. Heroin ranged from a low of about 13% in 1993, to a high of around 18% in 1988 and 1989. Marijuana fluctuated from 13% in 1989 to 19% in 1992.

Total expenditures for all illegal drugs has fallen in terms of dollars. The proportions spent for specific drugs have remained fairly stable. One might conclude that the dollar amount spent for any given drug should be falling as well. The problem with this generalization, however, is that even though the percentages of expenditures for a specific drug in any given year have remained fairly consistent, the actual dollars spent for that specific drug may or may not correlate with its respective percentage change. This is because of the interdependent relationship of percentages as a unit of measurement. For instance, although the expenditures for marijuana had the greatest percentage range (13-19%), the actual dollars spent were the same in 1989, 1991, and 1993 ($9.0 million).

Source Office of National Drug Control Policy. Executive Office of the President of the United States. *National Drug Control Strategy, Strengthening Communities' Response to Drugs and Crime, February 1995.* Washington, D.C.: U.S. Government Printing Office, [1995], table B-14, p. 145. Primary source: Abt Associates, Inc., *What America's Users Spend on Illegal Drugs, 1988-93, February 1995.*

Contact Executive Office of the President of the United States, Office of National Drug Control Policy, Washington, D.C. 20500; (202) 395-6700.

Retail Prices for Cocaine: 1988–93

The estimated prices per gram of pure cocaine in the U.S. from 1988–93.

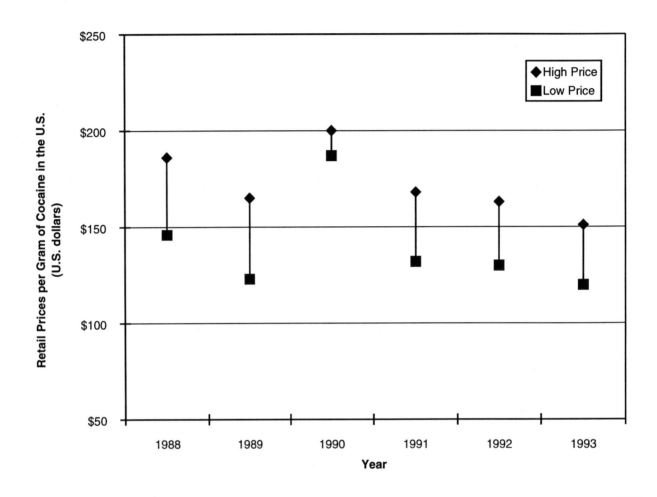

	1988	1989	1990	1991	1992	1993
High price	$186	$165	$200	$168	$163	$151
Low price	$146	$123	$187	$132	$130	$120

Comments Between 1988 and 1993, the estimated price for a pure gram of cocaine generally declined (in constant 1994 dollars), as shown by the graph. Moreover, the overall price range (the difference between the high and low prices) decreased as well, with a significant price range constriction occurring in 1990.

In the legal economy, when the supply of a product decreases (relative to a stable level of demand), then the product becomes more scarce, allowing producers to raise prices. This concept has also been applied to the illicit drug trade. Part of the economic strategy to fight the drug problem is the belief that increasing drug prices will discourage individual consumption. According to the Drug Enforcement Administration (DEA), in 1993 the price of cocaine was low, while the purity was high, even though coca cultivation declined in 1992 and 1993.

One explanation for this inconsistency may be that overall cocaine availability may not have actually decreased in 1993, especially if the decrease in cultivation was planned and production was supplemented by increasing production elsewhere. Another possibility may be that cocaine is being stockpiled in order to maintain a steady supply by allowing producers to cover a short-term market shortage. Still another possible explanation for the decreasing price may come from an increasing amount of competition among a larger number of drug sellers pursuing a shrinking customer base of drug users. This increased competition forces sellers to absorb higher costs of doing business, which means reduced profits.

Source Office of National Drug Control Policy. Executive Office of the President of the United States. *National Drug Control Strategy, Strengthening Communities' Response to Drugs and Crime, February 1995.* Washington, D.C.: U.S. Government Printing Office, [1995], table 4-2, p. 46. Primary source: Abt Associates, Inc., *What America's Users Spend on Illegal Drugs, 1988–93*, February 1995.

Contact Executive Office of the President of the United States, Office of National Drug Control Policy, Washington, D.C. 20500; (202) 395-6700.

Retail Prices of Heroin: 1988–93

The estimated prices per gram of pure heroin in the U.S. from 1988–93.

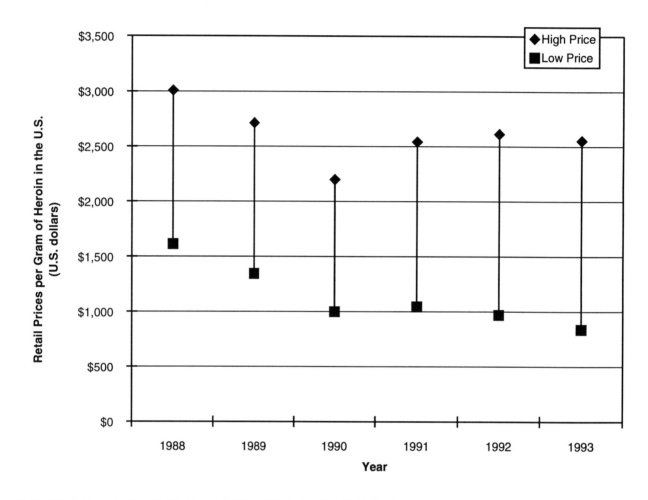

	1988	1989	1990	1991	1992	1993
High price	$3,007	$2,713	$2,199	$2,543	$2,614	$2,553
Low price	$1,612	$1,343	$997	$1,046	$968	$837

Comments

Heroin prices declined throughout the 1980s. Between 1988 and 1993 the estimated price for a gram of pure heroin powder continued to fall (in constant 1994 dollars) and is currently at its lowest level ever. For heroin, the price per pure gram was calculated by dividing the price by the average purity percentage for seized and purchased samples. Along with these lower prices has come an increase in heroin purity. This indicates that there is currently an abundant supply of heroin in the U.S. The overall price range (the difference between the high and low prices), however, has shown a trend of increasing, except for a significant price range constriction occurring in 1989–1990.

A typical heroin user pays about $1.70 per milligram for heroin which is about 30% pure. The increased supply and purity of heroin in the U.S. now enables users to smoke the drug rather than inject it. This fact alone may result in more heroin users. Some individuals would not use heroin at all if the only method of administration were by injection, mainly because of HIV infection among intravenous illicit drug users.

Source

Office of National Drug Control Policy. Executive Office of the President of the United States. *National Drug Control Strategy, Strengthening Communities' Response to Drugs and Crime, February 1995.* Washington, D.C.: U.S. Government Printing Office, [1995], p. *146.* Primary source: Abt Associates, Inc., *What America's Users Spend on Illegal Drugs, 1988–93*, February 1995.

Contact

Executive Office of the President of the United States, Office of National Drug Control Policy, Washington, D.C. 20500; (202) 395-6700.

Retail Price of Cocaine by Region: 1986-91

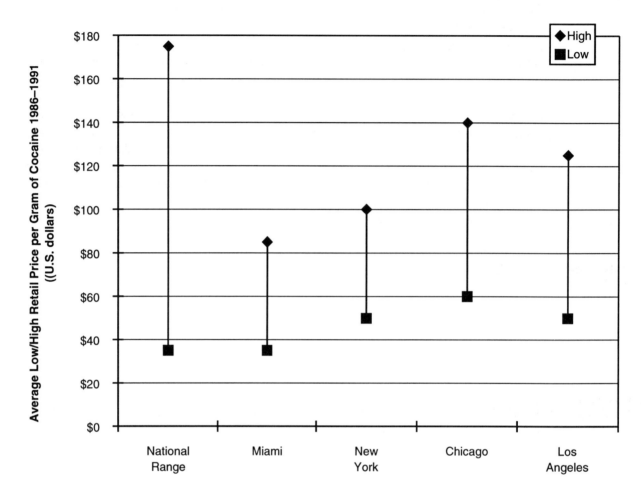

	1986	1987	1988	1989	1990	1991*
National range	$80-120	$80-120	$50-120	$35-125	$35-175	$40-175
Miami	50-60	50-60	55-85	50-80	35-80	60-70
New York	70-100	80-100	50-90	50-80	50-80	50-90
Chicago	100	100	75-100	70-100	60-100	100-140
Los Angeles	100	100	50-100	60-125	80-125	80-125

* First half of year only.

Comments Comparable to prices of legal products, the retail price for cocaine varies by location, and for many of the same reasons. First, the retail prices differ because of the various drug routes and distances involved from producer to distributor to end consumer. In addition, the local number of layers of distribution varies from place to place—the more distributors, the higher the price before the cocaine reaches the retail level. Local prices are also affected by shortages of drug supply due to wholesale and retail losses.

Local price changes may also occur because of costs passed on by various sellers. Buyers may also be willing to pay more for a specific type of cocaine from a particular nation. (This is much like brand loyalty in the legitimate market.) Finally, price changes may also reflect changes in the risks associated with dealing. However, these risks usually result in changes in purity rather in than cost to the retail buyer.

Source U.S. Department of Justice. Office of Justice Programs. Bureau of Justice Statistics. *Drugs, Crime, and the Justice System, A National Report from the Bureau of Justice Statistics, December 1992, NCJ-133652.* Washington, D.C.: U.S. Government Printing Office, [1992], p. 54. Primary source: Drug Enforcement Administration, *Illegal Drug Wholesale/Retail Prices Report, 1985 to March 1988* and *Illegal Drug Price/Purity Report, United States, Calendar Year 1988 through June 1991*, October 1991, p. 2.

Contact Drug Enforcement Administration, 600-700 Army Navy Dr., Arlington, VA 22202. Public Affairs: (202) 307-7977.

National Clearinghouse for Alcohol and Drug Information: (800) 729-6686.

Wholesale Prices for Marijuana: 1991

Wholesale prices per pound of marijuana according to country of origin,
showing high and low prices for each country.

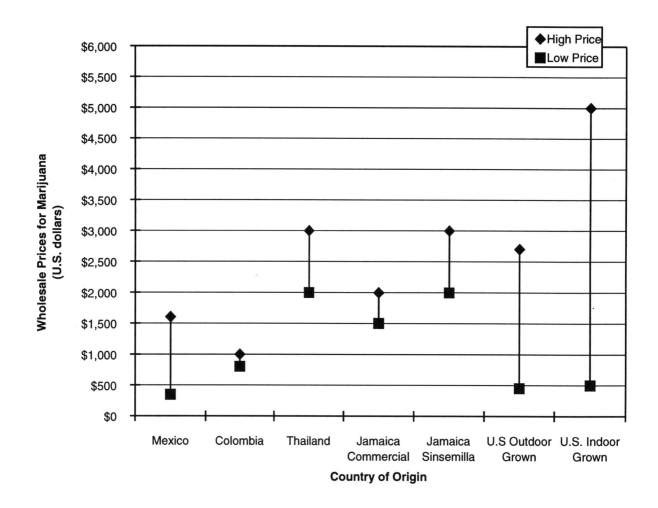

	Mexico	Colombia	Thailand	Jamaica Commercial Grade	Jamaica Sinsemilla	U.S. Outdoor Grown	U.S. Indoor Grown
High price	$1,600	$1,000	$3,000	$2,000	$3,000	$2,700	$5,000
Low price	$350	$800	$2,000	$1,500	$2,000	$450	$500

Comments

The wholesale price for marijuana can vary substantially depending on the drug's origin. Various factors—such as distance, distribution channels, risk associated with the illegal activity, and product quality and consistency—determine how much money will be paid for a pound of marijuana at the wholesale level.

As shown by the chart, such factors are less relevant to price ranges for marijuana from Colombia for example, but can lead to substantial price volatility for marijuana grown indoors in the U.S. In general, price increases of illegal drugs before they enter the U.S. are small relative to price increases after-

wards, mostly because risks to distributors and dealers rise significantly once the drug is in the U.S.

If, for example, a wholesale dealer of marijuana in the U.S. had the ability and desire to pay $2,000 per pound, then he or she could choose to buy a high-priced Jamaica commercial grade, low-priced Jamaica sinsemilla, Thailand marijuana, a fairly high-priced U.S. outdoor grown variety, or a relatively low-priced U.S. indoor grown variety. At $2,000 per pound, this figurative wholesale buyer would most likely not consider buying from Mexico or Colombia, since he would pay a higher price.

Source

U.S. Department of Justice. Office of Justice Programs. Bureau of Justice Statistics. *Drugs, Crime, and the Justice System, A National Report from the Bureau of Justice Statistics, December 1992, NCJ-133652.* Washington, D.C.: U.S. Government Printing Office, [1992], p. 54. Primary source: Drug Enforcement Administration, *From the Source to the Street: Mid-1991 Prices for Cannabis, Cocaine, and Heroin*, forthcoming, pp. 2 and 5–6.

Contact

Drug Enforcement Administration, 600-700 Army Navy Dr., Arlington, VA 22202. Public Affairs: (202) 307-7977. National Clearinghouse for Alcohol and Drug Information: (800) 729-6686.

Wholesale Cocaine Prices: 1991

Wholesale prices per kilogram of cocaine according to country of origin,
showing high and low prices for each country.

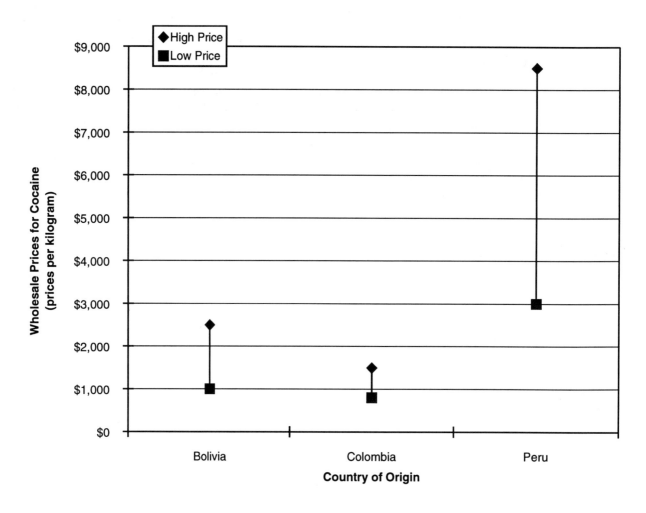

	Bolivia	Colombia	Peru
High price	$2,500	$1,500	$8,500
Low price	$1,000	$800	$3,000

Comments The wholesale price for cocaine can vary substantially depending on the drug's origin. Various factors—such as distance, distribution channels, risk associated with illegal activity, and product quality and consistency—determine the price of a kilogram of cocaine at the wholesale level. As shown by the chart, such factors are less relevant to price ranges for cocaine from Colombia and Bolivia, but are possibly more important cost factors for cocaine produced in Peru. In general, price increases of illegal drugs before they enter the U.S. are small relative to price increases afterwards, mainly because risks to distributors and dealers rise significantly once the drug is in the U.S.

Source U.S. Department of Justice. Office of Justice Programs. Bureau of Justice Statistics. *Drugs, Crime, and the Justice System, A National Report from the Bureau of Justice Statistics, December 1992, NCJ-133652*. Washington, D.C.: U.S. Government Printing Office, [1992], p. 54. Primary source: Drug Enforcement Administration, *From the Source to the Street: Mid-1991 Prices for Cannabis, Cocaine, and Heroin*, forthcoming, pp. 2 and 5–6.

Contact Drug Enforcement Administration, 600-700 Army Navy Dr., Arlington, VA 22202. Public Affairs: (202) 307-7977. National Clearinghouse for Alcohol and Drug Information: (800) 729-6686.

Costs to Society from Illegal Drug Use

The financial and potential opportunity costs to society as a result of illegal drug use.

Criminal Justice Expenditures on Drug-Related Crime	Health Care Costs	Lost Productivity Costs	Other Costs to Society
• Investigating robberies, burglaries, and thefts for drug money and adjudicating and punishing the offenders • Investigating assaults and homicides in the drug business (or by a drug user who has lost control) and adjudicating and punishing the offenders	• Injuries resulting from drug-related child abuse/neglect • Injuries from drug-related accidents • Injuries from drug-related crime • Other medical care for illegal drug users, including volunteer services and outpatient services, such as emergency room visits • Resources used in non-hospital settings	• Of drug-related accident victims • Of drug-related crime victims • Time away from work and homemaking to care for drug users and their dependents • Drug-related educational problems and school dropouts • Offenders incarcerated for drug-related or drug-defined crimes	• Loss of property values due to drug-related neighborhood crime • Property damaged or destroyed in fires, and in workplace and vehicular accidents • Agricultural resources devoted to illegal drug cultivation/production • Toxins introduced into the public air and water supplies by drug production • Workplace prevention programs such as drug testing and employee assistance programs • Averting behavior by potential victims of drug-related crime • Pain and suffering costs to illegal drug users and their families and friends

Comments Many of the social costs from illegal drug use can be quantified or estimated. There are other costs which are unavailable or which cannot be easily assigned a dollar value. Drug users lose income and the nation's economy suffers from lost productivity when drug users are unable to work as much, or as efficiently, as they could if they were not using drugs. When illegal drug users are put in prisons or are career criminals, they are unable or unwilling to work in the legitimate economy. Society also suffers from lost future output in the labor force because of premature death from drug use, from the violence associated with illegal drug distribution, or from AIDS transmitted by drug use.

Source U.S. Department of Justice. Office of Justice Programs. Bureau of Justice Statistics. *Drugs, Crime, and the Justice System, A National Report from the Bureau of Justice Statistics, December 1992, NCJ-133652*. Washington, D.C.: U.S. Government Printing Office, [1992], p. 127.

Contact Bureau of Justice Statistics Clearinghouse, Box 6000, Rockville, MD 20850; (800) 732-3277. Drugs & Crime Data Center & Clearinghouse, 1600 Research Blvd., Rockville, MD 20850; (800) 666-3332.

Emergency Room Episodes and Drug Use: 1988–93

Emergency room visits in which the use of a drug was mentioned. The term "drug mentions"
refers to each case; "drug episodes" refers to the number of people involved.

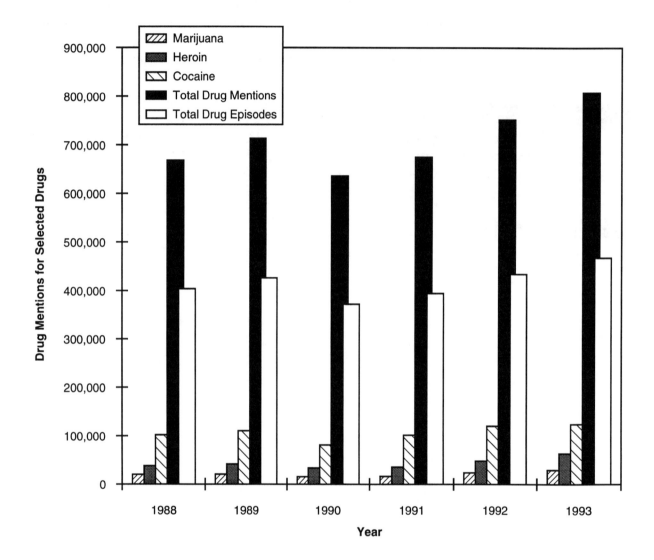

	1988	1989	1990	1991	1992	1993
Total marijuana mentions	19,962	20,703	15,706	16,251	23,997	29,166
Total heroin mentions	38,063	41,656	33,884	35,898	48,003	62,965
Total cocaine mentions	101,578	110,013	80,355	101,189	119,843	123,317
Total drug mentions	668,153	713,392	635,460	674,861	751,731	808,233
Total drug episodes (person cases)	403,578	425,904	371,208	393,968	433,493	466,897

Comments This chart helps illustrate the burdensome effects of drug use on the nation's medical system by showing the relationship between drug use and emergency room visits. Each episode represents a single hospital emergency room occurrence where the use of a drug was revealed or detected.

According to the information presented here, it is unclear whether the use of the drug directly caused the situation that necessitated an emergency room visit. Some episodes shown here may indeed be the result of a physiological trauma induced by drug use (especially for cocaine). Other episodes may have happened as a secondary hazard of drug abuse (e.g., accidents and assaults). Some of these episodes, specifically those caused by accidents, may also be linked to other emergency room incidents involving people who did not use illegal drugs.

Only three specific drugs are cited here—marijuana, heroin, and cocaine. The total number of drug mentions includes those three, in addition to all other drugs. The difference between the number of drug mentions and the number of drug episodes is that the two use different units of measurement. The category "total drug mentions" measures each occurrence as a case. "Total drug episodes" measures the number of people involved. A single individual may account for more than one drug mention at any given time.

According to the statistics portrayed in the chart, the annual number of emergency room drug mentions (as measured by the vertical scale on the left) rose overall during 1988-93, even though the level was down slightly in 1990 and 1991 from 1989. The mentions for the three specific drugs generally parallel the overall trend during those same years. The number of cocaine mentions closely parallels the total trend, while the number of heroin mentions proportionally has risen faster than the others since 1990.

Source Office of National Drug Control Policy. Executive Office of the President of the United States. *National Drug Control Strategy, Strengthening Communities' Response to Drugs and Crime, February 1995*. Washington, D.C.: U.S. Government Printing Office, [1995], table B-8, p. 143. Primary source: National Institute on Drug Abuse 1988-91, Drug Abuse Warning Network, and Substance Abuse and Mental Health Services Administration 1992-93.

Contact U.S. Department of Health and Human Services, Public Health Service, Substance Abuse and Mental Health Services Administration, National Institute on Drug Abuse, 5600 Fishers Lane, Rockville, MD 20857; (301) 443-6487. Public Relations: (301) 443-1124. National Clearinghouse For Alcohol and Drug Information: (800) 729-6686.

Drug-Induced Deaths by Gender: 1979–92

Deaths by drug-induced causes, except accidents and murders, by gender of the deceased.

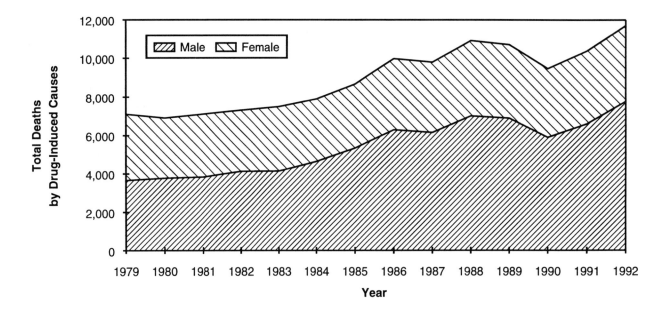

Year	Female	Male
1979	3,445	3,656
1980	3,129	3,771
1981	3,271	3,835
1982	3,180	4,130
1983	3,347	4,145
1984	3,252	4,640
1985	3,321	5,342
1986	3,692	6,284
1987	3,650	6,146
1988	3,913	7,004
1989	3,815	6,895
1990	3,566	5,897
1991	3,795	6,593
1992	3,937	7,766

Comments

Every year the Centers for Disease Control and Prevention (CDC) tabulates mortality (death) statistics for the U.S., including deaths caused directly by drug and alcohol use. These statistics, however, do not include accidents and homicides. The CDC defines drug-induced deaths by the following causes: drug psychoses; drug dependence; nondependent use of drugs (not including alcohol and tobacco); accidental poisonings by drugs, medicaments, and biologicals; suicide by drugs, medicaments, and biologicals; assault from poisoning by drugs and medicaments; and poisonings by drugs, medicaments, and biologicals which are undetermined, whether accidentally or purposely inflicted.

Source

U. S. Department of Health and Human Services. Public Health Service. Centers for Disease Control and Prevention. National Center for Health Statistics. "Advance Report of Final Mortality Statistics, 1992", *Monthly Vital Statistic Report*. 43, No. 6, suppl., [1995]: table 20, p. 59.

Contact

U.S. Department of Health and Human Services, Public Health Service, Centers for Disease Control and Prevention, National Center for Health Stastistics, 6525 Belcrest Rd., Hyattsville, MD 20782; (301) 436-8500. The National Center for Health Statistics maintains a World-Wide Web server at http://www.cdc.gov/nchswww/nchshome.htm

Reasons for Emergency Room Visits: 1993

Reported percentage giving reasons for drug-related emergency room contact.

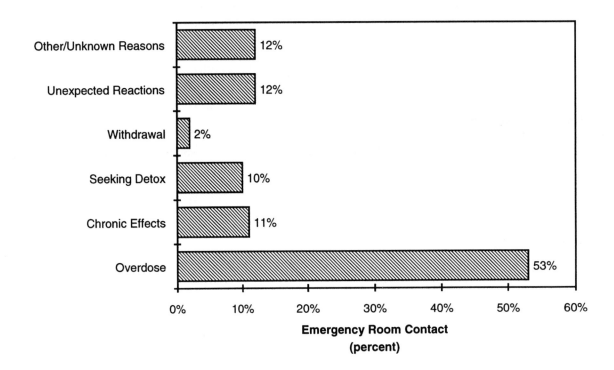

Reason	Percentage
Overdose	53%
Chronic effects	11%
Seeking detox	10%
Withdrawal	2%
Unexpected reactions	12%
Other/unknown reasons	12%

Comments This chart shows the most frequently given reasons for a drug-related emergency room visit. In 1993 there were 466,900 drug-related hospital emergency room episodes reported to the Drug Abuse Warning Network (DAWN). This represented a rate of 204 drug-related visits per 100,000 of the U.S. total population. This figure is up 22% from the rate of 167 per 100,000 population in 1990.

About one-half of all episodes involved the use of more than one drug. Of episodes involving the use of more than one drug, over half were caused by a drug overdose.

A drug-related hospital emergency room episode can represent a valuable opportunity for referring drug abusers to appropriate treatment programs. However, a lack of drug treatment facilities can prevent hospitals from helping drug users currently in their care. Furthermore, many persons involved in drug-related emergency room incidents may not be willing to enter treatment for substance abuse.

Source Office of National Drug Control Policy. Executive Office of the President of the United States. *National Drug Control Strategy, Strengthening Communities' Response to Drugs and Crime, February 1995.* Washington, D.C.: U.S. Government Printing Office, [1995], p. 36. Primary source: Substance Abuse and Mental Health Services Administration, National Institute on Drug Abuse, Drug Abuse Warning Network, 1993.

Contact U.S. Department of Health and Human Services, Public Health Service, Substance Abuse and Mental Health Services Administration, National Institute on Drug Abuse, 5600 Fishers Lane, Rockville, MD 20857; (301) 443-6487. Public Relations: (301) 443-1124. National Clearinghouse for Alcohol and Drug Information: (800) 729-6686.

Census of Clients in Alcohol and/or Drug Abuse Treatment: 1980–92

Total number of clients in alcohol and/or drug abuse treatment programs.

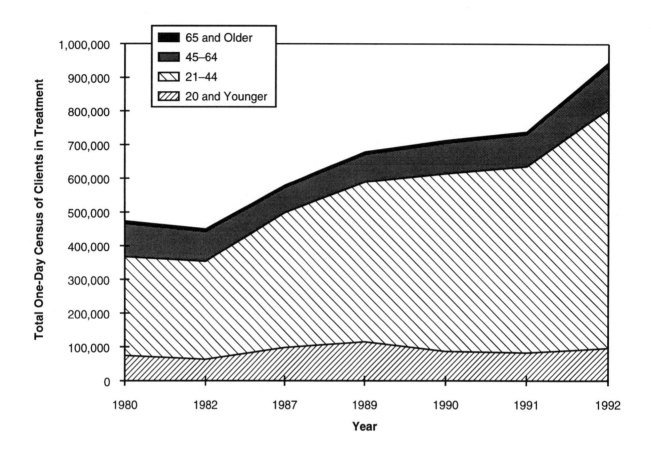

	1980	1982	1987	1989	1990	1991	1992
20 and younger	74,451	63,115	97,677	114,818	86,326	82,242	95,773
21–44	292,331	289,935	400,119	474,210	527,815	553,067	710,877
45–64	99,580	89,274	74,738	82,191	91,401	95,598	129,275
65 and older	7,194	6,734	6,557	7,134	7,214	7,464	8,954
Unknown	—	—	33,205	56,602	55,073	73,448	—
TOTAL	473,556	449,058	612,296	734,955	767,829	811,819	944,880

Comments This chart demonstrates the general age characteristics of individuals in alcohol and/or drug abuse treatment. The chart shows trends for the years 1980–92. The chart indicates that most of the individuals in alcohol and/or drug abuse treatment programs are between the ages of 21 and 44. All other age groups combined make up the minority of those involved in the treatment programs.

The overall trend of these statistics indicates that the total number of individuals in alcohol and/or drug abuse treatment programs In 1980, 473,556 persons were in treatment. By 1992, that number had increased 50% to 944,880. Again, the largest increase occurred in the 21–44 age group. In 1980, they represented 61% of all people in treatment, By 1992, they represented 75%.

Source Office of National Drug Control Policy. Executive Office of the President of the United States. *National Drug Control Strategy, Strengthening Communities' Response to Drugs and Crime, February 1995.* Washington, D.C.: U.S. Government

Printing Office, [1995], table B-10, p. 144. Primary source: National Institute on Drug Abuse, National Drug and Alcoholism Treatment Unit Survey, and National Institute on Alcohol Abuse and Alcoholism.

Contact U.S. Department of Health and Human Services, Public Health Service, Substance Abuse and Mental Health Services Administration, National Institute on Drug Abuse, 5600 Fishers Lane, Rockville, MD

20857; (301) 443-6487. Public Relations: (301) 443-1124. National Clearinghouse for Alcohol and Drug Information: (800) 729-6686.

Drug Abuse Treatment: 1989–96

Comparison of persons treated for drug abuse and those remaining to be treated, according to the number of treatment slots available.

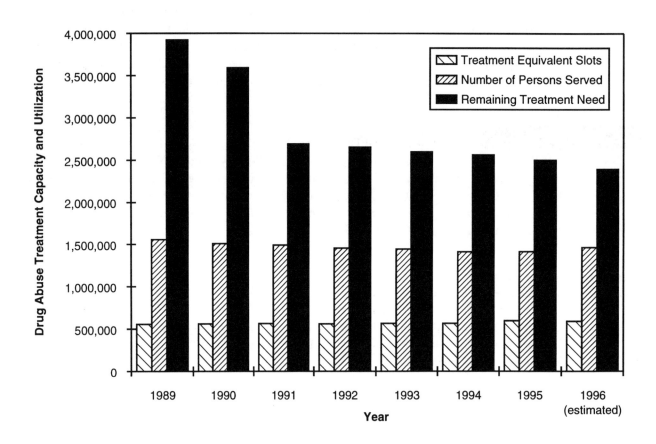

	1989	1990	1991	1992	1993	1994	1995	1996
Treatment equivalent slots	556,000	559,000	563,000	560,000	566,000	565,000	596,000	590,000
Number of persons served	1,557,000	1,509,000	1,491,000	1,455,000	1,443,000	1,412,000	1,413,000	1,460,000
Remaining treatment need	3,922,000	3,593,000	2,691,000	2,653,000	2,597,000	2,562,000	2,499,000	2,390,000
Percent of treatment goal received	47.0%	49.6%	56.4%	56.2%	56.7%	56.6%	57.8%	60.6%

Comments The figures presented here include only Substance Abuse and Mental Health Services Administration and National Institute on Drug Abuse in the federal estimates. Some of the federal agencies that provide substance abuse treatment, but are excluded from these estimates include the Departments of Veterans Affairs, Justice, Housing and Urban Development, and Defense, among others.

According to the figures presented, since 1989 the number of treatment slots has gradually increased every year (except 1994), peaking in 1995, before falling to an estimated 590,000 for 1996. The number of persons served, however, has steadily declined every year, from 1989 to 1994; this trend reversed in 1995 as the number of persons served is esti-

mated to grow to 1,460,000 for 1996. The larger number of persons remaining to be treated (as measured by the scale on the right) fell sharply from 1989 to 1991, but has only declined modestly since that time. With the exception of 1994, the proportion of the treatment goal that has been accomplished has risen every year.

If one only examines the number of treatment slots compared with the number of persons served, it might appear that there is a severe shortage of treatment slots. On the other hand, if only the percent of treatment goal received and the number of persons remaining to be treated are examined, then a more favorable observation can be made regarding this same problem.

Source Office of National Drug Control Policy. Executive Office of the President of the United States. *National Drug Control Strategy, Strengthening Communities' Response to Drugs and Crime, February* *1995.* Washington, D.C.: U.S. Government Printing Office, [1995], table B-9, p. 143. Primary source: U.S. Department of Health and Human Services.

Contact U.S. Department of Health and Human Services, Public Health Service, Substance Abuse and Mental Health Services Administration, National Institute on Drug Abuse, 5600 Fishers Lane, Rockville, MD 20857; (301) 443-6487. Public Relations: (301) 443-1124. National Clearinghouse for Alcohol and Drug Information: (800) 729-6686.

Drug Treatment Costs: 1989

Drug treatment costs according to funding source (in $ thousands) and percent of total funding.

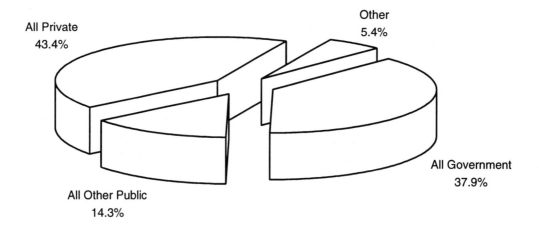

Funding Source	Thousands of Dollars	Percent
All government	**654,272**	**37.9**
Federal	53,230	3.1
State-local total	601,042	34.8
State	*436,738*	*25.3*
Local	*91,418*	*5.3*
Fee for service	*72,886*	*4.2*
All other public	**246,256**	**14.3**
Welfare	63,841	3.7
Third party	182,414	10.6
All private	**731,585**	**42.4**
Donations	32,651	1.9
Third party	505,398	29.3
Client fees	193,535	11.2
Other	**93,962**	**5.4**
TOTAL*	**$1,726,074**	**100.0**

* Detail does not add to total due to rounding.

Comments The Alcohol, Drug Abuse, and Mental Health Administration (ADAMHA), a branch of the U.S. Department of Health and Human Services, annually surveys private and public drug and alcohol treatment units and facilities. The survey is called the National Drug Treatment Unit Survey (NDATUS). The purpose of the survey is to assess the total cost of drug treatment and to determine how these costs are funded.

According to the survey, the estimated costs for drug treatment in the U.S. amounted to nearly $1.73 billion in 1989. However, this amount was believed to have been underestimated for several reasons. First, some 22% of known drug and alcohol treatment and prevention units did not respond to the NDATUS. Secondly, about 30% of all drug treatment units that did respond did not provide data regarding drug treatment funding. Also, some units did not report data for all their funding sources. Finally, no estimate was made for the funding of nonresponding facilities.

According to the information presented by the NDATUS, private sources provided the largest portion of funding for drug treatment costs (43.4%). Government sources provided 37.9% of the funding. Drug treatment costs averaged about $1,950 per client in 1989, with costs ranging from $338 per client for outpatient detoxification to $6,721 per client for inpatient hospital drug-free treatment.

Source U.S. Department of Justice. Office of Justice Programs. Bureau of Justice Statistics. *Drugs, Crime, and the Justice System, A National Report from the Bureau of Justice Statistics, December 1992, NCJ-133652.* Washington, D.C.: U.S. Government Printing Office, [1992], p. 133. Primary source: Alcohol, Drug Abuse, and Mental Health Administration (ADAMHA), *National Drug and Alcoholism Treatment Unit Survey (NDATUS): 1989 Main Findings Report*, 1990, table 46.

Contact U.S. Department of Health and Human Services, Alcohol, Drug Abuse, and Mental Health Administration, 5600 Fishers Lane, Rockville, MD 20857; (301) 443-3875.

tobacco

Per Capita Yearly Consumption of Cigarettes: 1900–94

Shows the average number of cigarettes smoked for each person in the U.S. (per capita)
18 years or older from 1900 to 1994.

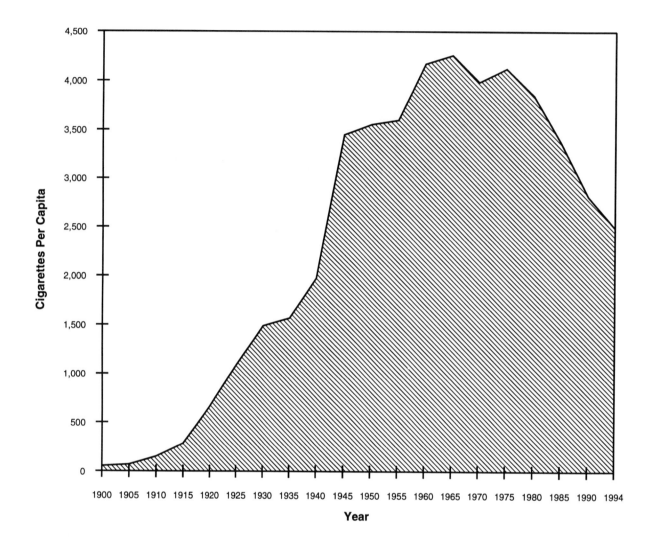

Comments This table shows consumption trends of manufactured cigarettes in the U.S. since the beginning of this century. Yearly consumption per adult (aged 18 and older) stood at just 54 cigarettes in 1900, and peaked at 4,345 in 1963, before gradually falling to 2,493 by 1994. With minor exceptions, per capita consumption increased steadily from 1900 to 1963.

Cigarette consumption got a boost in World War I (1917–1918) when the U.S. government liberally, and freely, supplied cigarettes to its soldiers. This increase in consumption created increased production in the cigarette industry, and cigarette consumption increased dramatically throughout the 1920s. Consumption leveled off with the onset of the Great Depression in 1929, but picked up again in 1935. The most dramatic increases in consumption coincided with America's entry into World War II. Cigarettes were highly valued by soldiers during WWII, and the increase in cigarette consumption reached its highest growth rates during the war years (1940–1945). One can assume that many Americans smoked their first cigarette while serving in the U.S. military. One can also assume that most continued to smoke after the war was over, for although the growth in cigarette consumption leveled off after the war, it did not decline.

The upward trend did not reverse until 1964. It was then that the U.S. Surgeon General issued his preliminary warning against the hazards of smoking. Since that announcement, consumption has steadily declined, with rebounds occurring in 1965–66 and 1971–73. Today, the per capita consumption is equivalent to that of 1942.

Source U.S. Department of Health and Human Services. Public Health Service. Centers for Disease Control and Prevention. "Surveillance for Selected Tobacco-Use Behaviors—United States, 1900–1994," *Morbidity and Mortality Weekly Report* 43, No. SS-3, [1994] pp. 6–7.

Contact Department of Health and Human Services, Public Health Service, Centers for Disease Control and Prevention, Atlanta, GA 30333. For inquiries about the *Morbidity and Mortality Weekly Report*, call (404) 332-4555. The CDC also maintains a World-Wide Web server at http://www.cdc.gov/.

Cigarette Smokers by State, 35 Years Old and Over: 1990

State-by-state percentage estimates of men and women cigarette smokers,
in age groups 35–64 and 65 and over, in 1990

State	Men 35–64	Women 35–64	Men ≥ 65	Women ≥ 65
Alabama	31.1	22.9	15.0	6.2
Alaska	33.3	24.5	17.8	13.2
Arizona	24.0	21.0	11.0	10.1
Arkansas	35.9	29.8	16.4	6.7
California	21.8	21.7	16.8	16.6
Colorado	24.2	26.4	12.5	11.4
Connecticut	27.4	22.9	11.8	12.0
Delaware	23.7	28.0	11.3	8.4
District of Columbia	30.4	21.0	21.2	6.8
Florida	33.7	21.6	17.4	13.1
Georgia	34.8	25.9	19.4	13.0
Hawaii	26.5	20.4	12.1	7.5
Idaho	23.7	20.8	12.5	11.8
Illinois	34.0	23.9	17.0	17.7
Indiana	33.1	26.4	16.8	11.7
Iowa	28.2	22.0	12.1	8.4
Kansas	30.7	18.7	14.2	6.7
Kentucky	39.7	29.0	19.1	11.3
Louisiana	32.7	24.7	14.9	8.6
Maine	33.2	24.3	17.0	12.7
Maryland	27.5	20.6	15.2	13.5
Massachusetts	28.2	20.1	16.5	15.3
Michigan	34.1	28.2	17.2	11.7
Minnesota	24.6	23.1	12.3	7.9
Mississippi	33.3	21.3	20.8	11.3
Missouri	31.9	23.6	14.9	11.2
Montana	25.2	25.1	12.2	15.6
Nebraska	33.3	25.5	20.9	7.9
Nevada	38.4	30.1	15.0	12.1
New Hampshire	25.2	21.5	16.3	14.5
New Jersey	28.8	25.1	13.0	15.1
New Mexico	22.8	25.1	15.7	11.7
New York	23.1	30.2	10.6	12.6
North Carolina	31.2	29.3	20.6	9.5
North Dakota	26.5	26.5	11.8	4.7
Ohio	30.3	27.7	9.1	12.9
Oklahoma	30.5	30.8	19.5	12.2

[Continued]

Cigarette Smokers by State: 35 Years Old and Over

[Continued]

State	Men 35–64	Women 35–64	Men ≥ 65	Women ≥ 65
Oregon	27.7	22.1	11.3	13.7
Pennsylvania	27.7	25.1	10.8	13.3
Rhode Island	28.5	26.4	18.5	10.3
South Carolina	39.4	24.8	26.0	13.6
South Dakota	25.8	21.8	18.3	9.9
Tennessee	33.0	28.4	25.1	12.1
Texas	27.0	25.9	18.3	14.9
Utah	25.2	14.6	10.8	7.3
Vermont	26.1	20.9	11.3	10.0
Virginia	28.7	24.7	16.3	14.4
Washington	26.7	19.9	15.7	15.5
West Virginia	32.7	26.2	18.3	16.4
Wisconsin	28.1	26.4	10.0	9.7
Wyoming	28.2	27.6	20.1	19.1

* The survey utilized the 1990 Behavioral Risk Factor Surveillance System for 44 states and the District of Columbia and the 1989 *Current Population Survey* of the U.S. Bureau of the Census for Alaska, Arkansas, Kansas, Nevada, New Jersey, and Wyoming.

Comments   The prevalence of smoking among middle-aged and older American adults varies greatly from state to state. However, in all cases, men are more likely than women to smoke. State-specific estimates regarding the frequency of cigarette smoking among persons aged 35–64 years ranged from 21.8% (California) to 39.7% (Kentucky) for men, and from 14.6% (Utah) to 30.8% (Oklahoma) for women. For persons 65 and older, the prevalence varied from 9.1% (Ohio) to 26.0% (South Carolina) for men and from 4.7% (North Dakota) to 19.1% (Wyoming) for women. In all cases the data would seem to suggest that people tend to smoke less as they grow older.

Source   U.S. Department of Health and Human Services. Public Health Service. Centers for Disease Control and Prevention. "Surveillance for Smoking-Attributable Mortality and Years of Potential Life Lost, by State—United States, 1990." *Morbidity and Mortality Report* 43, No. SS-1, (1994) pp. 1–8.

Contact   Department of Health and Human Services, Public Health Service, Centers for Disease Control and Prevention, Atlanta, GA 30333. For inquiries about the *Morbidity and Mortality Weekly Report*, call (404) 332-4555. The CDC also maintains a World-Wide Web server at http://www.cdc.gov/.

Cigarette Smokers by Race, Education, Age, and Income: 1992

Percentages of men and women 18 and older who were smokers in 1992. The data are grouped
by race/ethnic group, years of education completed, age group, and socioeconomic class
(above or below poverty level or unknown)

	Men (%)	Men's Margin of Error	Women (%)	Women's Margin of Error
By Race/Ethnicity				
White	28.6	(±0.9%)	25.9	(±0.8%)
Black	32.3	(±2.8%)	24.1	(±2.0%)
Hispanic	23.6	(±2.9%)	18.0	(±2.3%)
American Indian/Alaskan Native	39.0	(±10.4%)	39.8	(±6.8%)
Asian/Pacific Islander	26.3	(±6.4%)	4.0	(±2.0%)
By Education Level (years)				
< 12	36.9	(±1.8%)	27.5	(±1.4%)
12	34.4	(±1.3%)	28.2	(±1.1%)
13–15	25.2	(±1.7%)	23.1	(±1.4%)
16	16.2	(±1.4%)	14.6	(±1.4%)
By Age Group (years)				
18–24	28.0	(±2.5%)	24.9	(±2.0%)
25–44	32.8	(±1.2%)	28.8	(±1.1%)
45–64	28.6	(±1.5%)	26.1	(±1.3%)
> 65	16.1	(±1.6%)	12.4	(±1.1%)
By Socioeconomic Status*				
At/above poverty level	27.1	(±0.9%)	23.8	(±0.8%)
Below poverty level	39.7	(±2.6%)	31.7	(±1.7%)
Unknown	33.8	(±2.7%)	22.1	(±1.8%)
TOTALS	28.6	(±0.8%)	24.6	(±0.7%)

* As prescribed by the Office of Management and Budget.

Comments

Although the proportion of adult smokers declined from 1965 to 1990, in 1992 an estimated 48 million adults (26.5%) in the U.S. were smokers. Of these, about 22.1% were daily smokers, and 4.4% were some-day (or intermittent) smokers.

The Centers for Disease Control and Prevention (CDC) continually monitors the use of tobacco within the U.S., using the National Health Interview Survey—Cancer Control and Epidemiology Supplements (NHIS-CCES). According to the survey, smoking was more common among men for most demographic groups. Among ethnic groups, the prevalence of smoking was most common for American Indian/Alaskan Natives and lowest among Asian/Pacific Islanders. Smoking declined with increasing levels of education, and was highest for persons living below the poverty level.

For the first time since 1983, the prevalence of smoking in 1992 among persons aged 18–24 years did not decrease. Some believe the reason for the reversal in this trend is from the steady growth in the popularity of inexpensive discount cigarettes and the $4.6 billion in advertising and promotional expenditures by the tobacco companies in 1991 (up 16% from 1990).

This table shows not only the percentages of smokers, but also gives a margin of error, or *confidence interval*, to further indicate how reliable that percentage might be to describe the whole population. For example, the prevalence of smoking for white males was estimated at 28.6% (with a confidence interval of ±0.9%). This means that the actual rate for white males could be as low as 27.7% or as high as 29.5%.

Source

U.S. Department of Health and Human Services. Public Health Service. Centers for Disease Control and Prevention. "Cigarette Smoking Among Adults—United States, 1992, and Changes in the Definition of Current Cigarette Smoking," *Morbidity and Mortality Weekly Report* 43 No. 19, (1994) pp. 342–346.

Contact

Department of Health and Human Services, Public Health Service, Centers for Disease Control and Prevention, Atlanta, GA 30333. For inquiries about the *Morbidity and Mortality Weekly Report*, call (404) 332-4555. The CDC also maintains a World-Wide Web server at http://www.cdc.gov/.

Women Smokers Aged 18–44: 1987–92

Percentages of women cigarette smokers aged 18–44, listed by years of education completed
and by socioeconomic class (above or below poverty level or unknown).
Results of a U.S. National Health Interview Survey, 1987–92.

	1987	1988	1989	1990	1991	1992
TOTAL	29.6%	28.8%	27.6%	25.6%	26.7%	26.9%
Education (yrs)						
< 12	46.5	45.9	42.7	40.6	40.5	40.2
12	33.7	32.7	31.2	31.1	32.0	31.9
13–15	24.7	24.7	25.9	20.6	22.8	24.0
≥ 16	14.2	13.9	12.0	10.5	12.0	12.5
Socioeconomic Status						
At/above poverty level	28.3	27.2	26.4	23.6	25.3	24.7
Below poverty level	37.0	38.0	34.9	36.1	32.7	40.0
Unknown	31.1	31.9	28.9	30.4	31.0	24.7

Comments Women who smoke cigarettes have a greater risk of developing lung cancer, chronic obstructive pulmonary disease, and complications from oral contraceptive use. During pregnancy, cigarette smoking increases the risk for a low birthweight infant and infant mortality. In 1992, an estimated 14.3 million (26.9%) of all U.S. women aged 18–44 years were smokers. The prevalence of smoking among women in that age group fell substantially from 29.6% in 1987 to 25.6% in 1990, but increased to 26.7% in 1991. According to these statistics, smoking becomes less common among women of reproductive years with higher levels of education.

Source U.S. Department of Health and Human Services. Public Health Service. Centers for Disease Control and Prevention. "Cigarette Smoking Among Women of Reproductive Age—United States, 1987–1992." *Morbidity and Mortality Weekly Report* 43, No. 43, (1994) pp. 789–792.

Contact Department of Health and Human Services, Public Health Service, Centers for Disease Control and Prevention, Atlanta, GA 30333. For inquiries about the *Morbidity and Mortality Weekly Report*, call (404) 332-4555. The CDC also maintains a World-Wide Web server at http://www.cdc.gov/.

Cigarette Smoking by High School Seniors: 1975–94

Trends in cigarette smoking among high school seniors, according to frequency of use (in percent).
Shown by year, 1975–94.

Year	Half-Pack or More Daily	Daily Use	Past Month	Ever Used
1975	17.9	26.9	36.7	73.6
1976	19.2	28.8	38.8	75.4
1977	19.4	28.8	38.4	75.7
1978	18.8	27.5	36.7	75.3
1979	16.5	25.4	34.4	74.0
1980	14.3	21.3	30.5	71.0
1981	13.5	20.3	29.4	71.0
1982	14.2	21.1	30.0	70.1
1983	13.8	21.2	30.3	70.6
1984	12.3	18.7	29.3	69.7
1985	12.5	19.5	30.1	68.8
1986	11.4	18.7	29.6	67.6
1987	11.4	18.7	29.4	67.2
1988	10.6	18.1	28.7	66.4
1989	11.2	18.9	28.6	65.7
1990	11.3	19.1	29.4	64.4
1991	10.7	18.5	28.3	63.1
1992	10.0	17.2	27.8	61.8
1993	10.9	19.0	29.9	61.9
1994	11.2	19.4	31.2	62.0

Comments   Smoking by high school seniors has declined since the mid-1970s, according to survey statistics gathered each year by the National Institute on Drug Abuse. During the mid-1970s, nearly four of every five high school seniors surveyed had tried smoking cigarettes at some point in their lives. By the early 1990s, that proportion had fallen to three of every five. Since most adult smokers started smoking during their teens, examining such statistics can be useful in understanding long-term patterns and trends regarding smoking.

For example, of the high school seniors who had ever used cigarettes in 1975, about 25% reported smoking a half-pack or more daily. In 1994, that ratio had dropped to just 18%. This indicates that not only were fewer high school seniors trying cigarettes, but that the tendency for those who did try smoking to become heavy users was also declining.

The percent of high school seniors who reported using cigarettes within the past month remained more stable throughout the 1980s. However, after falling in the late 1970s, these percentages began to rise in 1993 and 1994. This trend may indicate a rising trend in casual smoking among some high school seniors; these casual users often become daily users.

Source   U.S. Department of Health and Human Services. Public Health Service. Substance Abuse and Mental Health Services Administration. National Institute on Drug Abuse. "Monitoring the Future Study, 1975–1994: National High School Senior Drug Abuse Survey 1994."

Contact   U.S. Department of Health and Human Services. Public Health Service. Substance Abuse and Mental Health Services Administration. National Institute on Drug Abuse, 5600 Fishers Lane, Rockville, MD 20857; (301) 443-6487.

Cigarette Smoking by Youths Aged 12–21: 1992

Percentage of smokers from ages 12 to 21 by status (current, former, experimenter or never) and by gender, 1992.

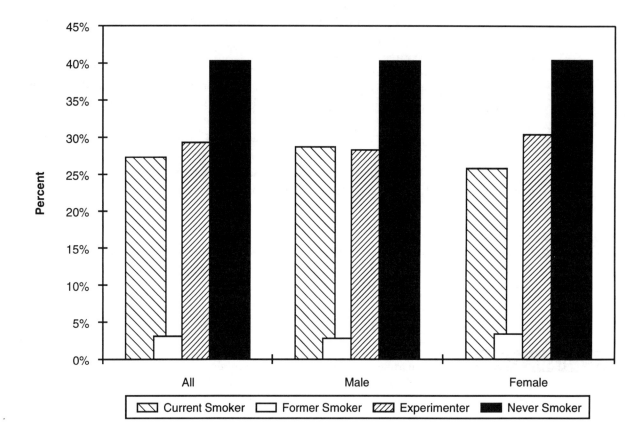

Status	All	Male	Female
Current smoker	27.3%	28.7%	25.8%
Former smoker	3.1%	2.8%	3.4%
Experimenter	29.3%	28.3%	30.4%
Never smoker	40.3%	40.3%	40.4%

Adolescents often develop behaviors that extend into adulthood. These bhaviors include cigarette smoking, a risky health behavior with long-term health consequences. Young people start smoking in an effort to bond with peers, improve their perceived social image, and appear independent and mature. Cigarette smoking almost always begins in the adolescent years, and smoking at early ages increases the risk of becoming ill or dying from causes attributable to smoking later in life.

A reduction in smoking among adolescents is one of the objectives established in the National Health Objectives for the Year 2000, by the Department of Health and Human Services. The information presented here was collected from the 1992 National Health Interview Survey of Youth Risk Behavior. Also included in the survey, but not reported here, are estimates among adolescents for several other unhealthy behaviors, including: drinking alcohol; consuming more than five alcoholic beverages in a row; using marijuana, cocaine, and smokeless tobacco; carrying weapons; physical fighting; sexual intercourse; failure to use a seat belt; lack of exercise; and consumption of fewer than five servings of fruits and vegetables per day.

This survey defines a current smoker as an adult who has smoked 100 cigarettes in his or her lifetime and who smokes "now," or an adolescent who has smoked at least one cigarette in the past thirty days.

Former smokers are youth who had smoked at least one cigarette every day for 30 days at some time in their lives, but have not smoked in the past month. Experimenters are youth who have had at least one or two puffs of a cigarette, but who have never smoked cigarettes every day for 30 days, and who have not used cigarettes in the past 30 days. "Never smokers" are youths who have never even had one or two puffs of a cigarette.

In 1992, about 29% of male and 26% of female youths were current smokers, and about 3% of each sex were former smokers. An estimated 28% of the male and 30% of the female youths had experimented with cigarettes, but had never smoked regularly. Approximately 40% of youths had never taken even a puff of a cigarette.

Source J.C. Willard and C.A. Schoenborn, "Relationship Between Cigarette Smoking and Other Unhealthy Behaviors Among Our Nation's Youth: United States, 1992." Advance data from vital and health statistics; No. 263. National Center for Health Statistics, 1995.

Contact Department of Health and Human Services, Public Health Service, Centers for Disease Control and Prevention, National Center for Health Statistics, 6525 Belcrest Rd., Hyattsville, MD 20782; (301) 436-8500.

Smokeless Tobacco Use by Teenagers: 1986–94

Percentage of surveyed 8th and 10th graders from 1991–94 and 12th graders from 1986–94
who used smokeless tobacco. Listed by frequency of use.

Percentage of surveyed 8th graders reporting smokeless tobacco use, 1991–94

Year	Use Daily	Used Within Past Month	Ever Used
1991	1.6	6.9	22.2
1992	1.8	7.0	20.7
1993	1.5	6.6	18.7
1994	1.9	7.7	19.9

Percentage of surveyed 10th graders reporting smokeless tobacco use, 1991–94

Year	Use Daily	Used Within Past Month	Ever Used
1991	3.3	10.0	28.2
1992	3.0	9.6	26.6
1993	3.3	10.4	28.1
1994	3.0	10.5	29.2

Percentage of surveyed 12th graders reporting smokeless tobacco use, 1986–94

Year	Use Daily	Used Within Past Month	Ever Used
1986	4.7	11.5	31.4
1987	5.1	11.3	32.2
1988	4.3	10.3	30.4
1989	3.3	8.4	29.2
1990*	—	—	—
1991*	—	—	—
1992	4.3	11.4	32.4
1993	3.3	10.7	31.0
1994	3.9	11.1	30.7

* No data available.

Comments   Smokeless tobacco (chewing tobacco and snuff) is another tobacco product commonly used by minors, but much less so than cigarettes. Among high school seniors who had tried smokeless tobacco, 73% typically did so by the 9th grade.

Statistics given in the report cited below, but not reported in the accompanying graph, indicated that the use of smokeless tobacco among young men has become more popular since the late 1970s. The prevalence of smokeless tobacco use by males aged 18–24 increased from 2.2% in 1970 to 10.1% in 1991. The rate for females in that age group remained at 0.2% from 1970 to 1991.

Since smokeless tobacco use among young men aged 18–24 increased so rapidly, their behavior may have affected the desire of males younger than 18 to try and use smokeless tobacco. The popularity of smokeless tobacco among men is especially high in West Virginia, Montana, and several southern states.

Source   U.S. Department of Health and Human Services. Public Health Service. Centers for Disease Control and Prevention. National Institute on Drug Abuse, "Monitoring the Future Study," 1994. "Surveillance for Selected Tobacco-Use Behaviors—United States, 1900–94," *Morbidity and Mortality Weekly Report* 43, No. SS-3, (1994).

Contact   Department of Health and Human Services, Public Health Service, Centers for Disease Control and Prevention, Atlanta, GA 30333. For inquiries about the *Morbidity and Mortality Weekly Report*, call (404) 332-4555. The CDC also maintains a World-Wide Web server at http://www.cdc.gov/.

Prevalence of Selected Reasons for Using Cigarettes: 1993

Percentage by age group and use history.
Results of Teenage Attitudes and Practices Survey, 1993

	Percent responding: "It relaxes or calms me"	Percent responding: "It's really hard to quit"
Total Cigarettes Smoked (lifetime use)		
10–18 years old		
< 20	30.5	8.2
21–98	48.7	21.1
> 100	66.8	63.1
19–22 years old		
< 20	18.1	3.8
21–98	39.5	10.4
> 100	69.2	64.8
Total Cigarettes Smoked (per day)		
10–18 years old		
≤ 5	57.3	61.5
6–15	69.7	74.4
≥ 16	75.4	71.1
19–22 years old		
≤ 5	39.6	34.6
6–15	72.4	73.4
≥ 16	82.6	78.8

Comments The nicotine contained in cigarettes and other forms of tobacco is an addictive substance. According to the Centers for Disease Control and Prevention (CDC), among adults in the U.S. who have ever smoked daily, 91.3% tried their first cigarette, and 77.0% became daily smokers before age 20. The CDC analyzed data from the 1993 Teenage Attitudes and Practices Survey (TAPS-II) to determine how nicotine addiction develops among persons aged 10 through 22.

Persons surveyed who reported having smoked cigarettes during the previous month were asked if they used tobacco because "it relaxes or calms me." They were also asked if they used tobacco because "it's hard to quit." Either answer indicates an influence of the properties of nicotine upon the brain. According to these statistics, as lifetime cigarette use increases, the gap between young people who smoke for relaxation and those who smoke because of 'addiction narrows. For example, for the 10–18 age group, for those individuals who had smoked 20 or fewer cigarettes in their lifetimes, 30.5% cited relaxation as a reason for smoking, while only 8.2% reported that they smoked because it was hard to quit. For those in that same age group who had smoked over 100 cigarettes, 66.8% did so for relaxation but 63.1% also reported smoking because it was hard to quit.

This observation is similar to other reports from the CDC indicating that adolescents initially try cigarettes because of advertising, social pressure, and curiosity. However, once the smoking becomes an established behavior, regular smokers are more likely than beginning smokers to report that they are addicted.

Source U.S. Department of Health and Human Services. Public Health Service. Centers for Disease Control and Prevention. "Reasons for Tobacco Use and Symptoms of Nicotine Withdrawal Among Adolescent and Young Adult Tobacco Users—United States, 1993." *Morbidity and Mortality Weekly Report* 43, No. 41, (1994) pp. 745–747.

Contact Department of Health and Human Services, Public Health Service, Centers for Disease Control and Prevention, Atlanta, GA 30333. For inquiries about the *Morbidity and Mortality Weekly Report*, call (404) 332-4555. The CDC also maintains a World-Wide Web server at http://www.cdc.gov/.

Nicotine Withdrawal Symptoms Reported by Teenagers: 1993

Percentage of tobacco users aged 10–22 who reported various nicotine withdrawal symptoms during their attempts to quit smoking. Listed by age group and frequency of use (number of days per month). Results of Teenage Attitudes and Practices Survey, 1993.

Age	Days Smoked per Month	Find It Hard to Concentrate	Feel Hungry More Often	Feel More Irritable	Strong Need/Urge to Smoke	Feel Restless	Feel Sad, Blue, Depressed	Any Indicator
10–18 Years	0	11.8	24.4	21.4	21.9	17.0	9.3	44.4
	1–14	22.8	35.4	36.5	36.3	30.3	17.9	66.0
	15–29	39.2	43.0	55.8	71.2	49.9	24.4	88.1
	30	46.1	49.0	77.0	81.6	62.6	28.6	93.9
19–22 Years	0	14.6	30.0	29.2	28.1	27.2	11.7	50.0
	1–14	16.9	40.5	32.5	43.8	32.2	11.5	68.7
	15–29	26.9	52.8	49.9	63.4	54.6	18.5	86.0
	30	47.3	50.5	70.9	78.1	60.8	23.1	91.7
10–22 Years	0	13.0	26.8	24.7	24.6	21.3	10.3	46.8
	1–14	20.5	37.4	35.0	39.2	31.0	15.4	67.0
	15–29	32.8	48.0	52.7	67.2	52.4	21.3	87.0
	30	46.8	49.9	73.5	79.6	61.6	25.5	92.4

Comments The CDC analyzed data from the 1993 Teenage Attitudes and Practices Survey (TAPS-II) to determine how nicotine addiction develops among persons aged 10 through 22. According to this survey, the likelihood of reporting symptoms of nicotine withdrawal increased in relation to frequency and intensity of use. Younger and older smokers were equally likely to report increasing nicotine withdrawal symptoms as exposure increased. For example, for the 10 to 18 year olds, only 44.4% of those who had not smoked within the past 30 days reported any of the withdrawal symptoms, while 93.3% of those who smoked during each of the preceding 30 days reported at least one indicator.

Source U.S. Department of Health and Human Services. Public Health Service. Centers for Disease Control and Prevention. "Reasons for Tobacco Use and Symptoms of Nicotine Withdrawal Among Adolescent and Young Adult Tobacco Users—United States, 1993." *Morbidity and Mortality Weekly Report* 43, No. 41, (1994) pp. 745–750.

Contact Department of Health and Human Services, Public Health Service, Centers for Disease Control and Prevention, Atlanta, GA 30333. For inquiries about the *Morbidity and Mortality Weekly Report*, call (404) 332-4555. The CDC also maintains a World-Wide Web server at http://www.cdc.gov/.

Costs of Medical Care for Smoking-Related Sickness: 1987

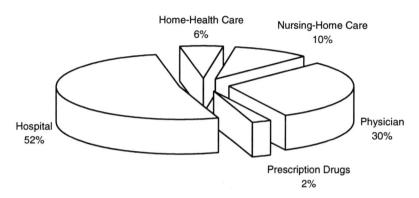

Amount (in $ millions) of total medical care spending on causes related to smoking, listed by age group and category of care.

Age Group (yrs)	Physician*	Prescription Drugs	Hospital	Home-Health Care**	Nursing-Home Care	TOTAL
19–64	$5,185	$224	$6,995	$371		$12,775
65 and over	$1,439	$303	$4,358	$861	$2,156	$9,117
TOTAL	$6,624	$527	$11,353	$1,232	$2,156	$21,892

* Includes hospital-based outpatient and emergency care in physicians' offices.
** Includes Medicare- and Medicaid-certified services and other reported services.

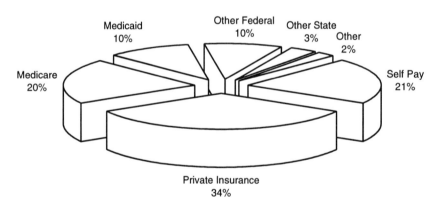

Amount (in $ millions) of total medical care spending on causes related to smoking, listed by age group and source of payment.

Age Group (yrs)	Self Pay	Private Insurance	Medicare	Medicaid	Other Federal	Other State	Other	TOTAL
19–64	$2,274	$6,119	$728	$1,086	$1,571	$600	$396	$12,775
65 and over	$2,325	$1,185	$3,756	$1,158	$520	$91	$82	$9,117
TOTAL*	$4,599	$7,304	$4,485	$2,244	$2,091	$692	$478	$21,892

* Numbers may not add to totals due to rounding.

Comments

About 400,000 deaths attributable to cigarette smoking occur each year in the U.S., and the costs associated with sickness attributable to smoking are sizable. In order to estimate the 1993 smoking-related costs for the selected categories of direct medical-care expenditures, the University of California and CDC analyzed data from the 1987 National Medical Expenditures Survey and from the Health Care Financing Administration.

According to the National Medical Expenditures Survey, the total medical-care expenditures for the five categories named in the pie chart were $308.7 billion, of which $21.9 billion (7.1%) was attributable to smoking. Hospital costs accounted for the largest share of all costs attributable to smoking ($11.4 billion), followed by physician care

and nursing-home care. Public funding (e.g., Medicaid, Medicare, and other state and federal sources) paid for 43.3% of the medical-care expenditures attributable to smoking. For persons aged 65 and older, public funding accounted for 60.6% of these costs, as compared to 31.2% for persons under age 65.

Cigarette smoking is the most prominent preventable cause of illness and premature death in the U.S., yet there are 48 million persons aged 18 and over who smoke. This group annually purchases 24 billion packs of cigarettes. Based on the 1987 survey, for each of the 24 billion packs of cigarettes sold in 1993, approximately $2.06 was spent on medical care attributable to smoking. Of the $2.06, about 89¢ was paid by taxpayers through public sources.

Source

U.S. Department of Health and Human Services. Public Health Service. Centers for Disease Control and Prevention. "Medical-Care Expenditures Attributable to Cigarette Smoking—United States, 1993," Centers for Disease Control and Prevention, *Morbidity and Mortality Weekly Report* 43, No. 26, (1994) pp. 469-473.

Contact

Department of Health and Human Services, Public Health Service, Centers for Disease Control and Prevention, Atlanta, GA 30333. For inquiries about the *Morbidity and Mortality Weekly Report*, call (404) 332-4555. The CDC also maintains a World-Wide Web server at http://www.cdc.gov/.

Potential Years of Life Lost Due to Smoking: 1990

Estimated totals of potential years of life lost due to smoking, listed by state and sex of smoker, 1990.

State	Male	Female	Total
Alabama	62,287	28,073	90,360
Alaska	4,711	2,009	6,720
Arizona	42,421	24,538	66,959
Arkansas	39,425	19,317	58,742
California	290,416	207,881	498,297
Colorado	29,800	19,200	49,000
Connecticut	35,943	24,592	60,535
Delaware	9,102	6,146	15,248
District of Columbia	13,512	7,660	21,172
Florida	206,881	121,310	328,191
Georgia	88,396	45,772	134,168
Hawaii	10,135	5,087	15,222
Idaho	9,052	5,656	14,708
Illinois	143,258	92,675	235,933
Indiana	79,155	44,429	123,584
Iowa	34,121	16,400	50,521
Kansas	28,713	13,827	42,540
Kentucky	61,404	33,198	94,602
Louisiana	62,828	32,058	94,886
Maine	16,879	10,540	27,419
Maryland	55,786	36,411	92,197
Massachusetts	68,822	48,818	117,640
Michigan	123,337	72,263	195,600
Minnesota	44,365	23,470	67,835
Mississippi	39,230	18,609	57,839
Missouri	79,112	43,024	122,136
Montana	8,741	5,750	14,491
Nebraska	20,060	9,015	29,075
Nevada	12,291	10,963	23,254
New Hampshire	11,675	7,318	18,993
New Jersey	90,653	61,120	151,773
New Mexico	12,710	8,446	21,156
New York	219,751	157,779	377,530
North Carolina	99,223	48,587	147,810
North Dakota	8,028	3,689	11,717
Ohio	140,831	90,666	231,497
Oklahoma	46,252	26,805	73,057
Oregon	36,425	22,792	59,217

[Continued]

Potential Years of Life Lost Due to Smoking: 1990

[Continued]

State	Male	Female	Total
Pennsylvania	168,532	103,307	271,839
Rhode Island	14,006	7,535	21,541
South Carolina	52,910	26,159	79,069
South Dakota	9,033	3,651	12,684
Tennessee	87,627	45,008	132,635
Texas	201,112	116,519	317,631
Utah	10,552	4,020	14,572
Vermont	7,042	3,589	10,631
Virginia	74,535	45,181	119,716
Washington	53,757	35,465	89,222
West Virginia	32,784	18,223	51,007
Wisconsin	54,529	31,816	86,345
Wyoming	4,509	2,789	7,298
Highest value	290,416	207,881	498,297
Lowest value	4,509	2,009	6,720
Median	42,421	24,538	66,959

Comments

In 1990, an estimated 415,226 smoking-attributable deaths occurred throughout the U.S. These deaths resulted in an estimated cumulative total of over 5 million years of potential life lost (or about 12 years per person). The numbers presented here do not include an estimated 3,000 additional deaths resulting from exposure to environmental smoke.

This large sum of years of potential life lost due to premature death from smoking has economic as well as social and personal implications.

Smoking-attributable deaths constantly erode the knowledge and skills base of human resources. Since smoking-attributable deaths often occur late in life, a significant proportion of fatalities will likely include those persons with the highest levels of career experience (having often achieved positions of leadership or authority). When the volume of these premature deaths is considered, it is possible to gain some insight into the effects of the physical risks of smoking on society and the economy at large.

Source

U.S. Department of Health and Human Services. Public Health Service. Centers for Disease Control and Prevention. "Surveillance for Smoking-Attributable Mortality and Years of Potential Life Lost, by State— United States, 1990." *Morbidity and Mortality Report* 43, No. SS-1, (1994) pp. 1–8.

Contact

Department of Health and Human Services, Public Health Service, Centers for Disease Control and Prevention, Atlanta, GA 30333. For inquiries about the *Morbidity and Mortality Weekly Report*, call (404) 332-4555. The CDC also maintains a World-Wide Web server at http://www.cdc.gov/.

Deaths Attributed to Smoking: 1990

Estimated totals of deaths due to smoking, listed by state and sex of smoker. Also listed are rates of death per 100,000 population, rank of state, and percent of all deaths in state due to smoking.

State	Male	Female	Total	Rate*	Rank†	Percent of All Deaths
Alabama	4,960	1,841	6,801	350.4	22	17.3
Alaska	290	112	402	398.2	46	18.4
Arizona	3,839	1,858	5,697	339.6	16	19.8
Arkansas	3,410	1,296	4,706	376.3	35	19.1
California	25,821	16,753	42,574	366.3	27	19.9
Colorado	2,658	1,513	4,171	331.4	13	19.3
Connecticut	3,337	2,025	5,362	325.7	12	19.4
Delaware	745	433	1,178	393.1	44	20.4
District of Columbia	874	413	1,287	444.7	50	17.6
Florida	18,865	9,731	28,596	357.5	24	21.3
Georgia	6,692	3,002	9,694	383.5	38	18.7
Hawaii	849	325	1,174	257.2	2	17.3
Idaho	865	439	1,304	293.2	4	17.5
Illinois	12,028	7,241	19,269	360.0	25	18.7
Indiana	6,924	3,326	10,250	394.3	45	20.7
Iowa	3,410	1,406	4,816	304.2	7	17.9
Kansas	2,728	1,100	3,828	300.8	6	17.2
Kentucky	5,127	2,322	7,449	428.7	47	21.2
Louisiana	4,829	2,058	6,887	388.2	40	18.3
Maine	1,508	868	2,376	389.4	42	21.4
Maryland	4,593	2,777	7,370	378.1	36	19.2
Massachusetts	6,132	4,298	10,430	345.3	17	19.6
Michigan	10,386	5,068	15,454	372.5	33	19.6
Minnesota	4,237	1,890	6,127	295.2	5	17.6
Mississippi	3,188	1,270	4,458	375.1	34	17.7
Missouri	6,907	3,270	10,177	383.8	39	20.2
Montana	856	457	1,313	334.2	15	19.1
Nebraska	1,965	710	2,675	321.0	11	18.1
Nevada	1,517	717	2,234	478.1	51	24.0
New Hampshire	1,036	619	1,655	349.3	20	19.5
New Jersey	7,734	4,871	12,605	334.1	14	17.9
New Mexico	1,097	644	1,741	287.7	3	16.4
New York	18,612	12,380	30,992	352.8	23	18.3
North Carolina	7,922	3,110	11,032	367.6	30	19.2
North Dakota	790	241	1,031	308.2	9	18.2
Ohio	11,421	6,693	18,114	347.7	19	18.3

[Continued]

Deaths Attributed to Smoking: 1990

[Continued]

State	Male	Female	Total	Rate*	Rank†	Percent of All Deaths
Oklahoma	4,132	2,006	6,138	390.4	43	20.2
Oregon	3,393	1,833	5,226	369.3	31	20.8
Pennsylvania	14,576	8,048	22,624	346.8	18	18.6
Rhode Island	1,250	631	1,881	350.3	21	19.6
South Carolina	3,928	1,691	5,619	380.1	37	18.9
South Dakota	877	298	1,175	307.9	8	18.6
Tennessee	7,146	3,068	10,214	442.1	49	22.1
Texas	16,705	8,747	25,452	389.1	41	20.3
Utah	940	288	1,228	218.0	1	13.4
Vermont	617	296	913	363.3	26	19.9
Virginia	5,926	3,311	9,237	366.6	28	19.2
Washington	4,892	2,898	7,790	367.4	29	21.0
West Virginia	2,831	1,390	4,221	433.6	48	21.8
Wisconsin	4,995	2,625	7,650	313.3	10	17.8
Wyoming	419	240	659	371.0	32	20.6
Highest value	25,821	16,753	42,574	478.1	—	24.0
Lowest value	290	112	402	218.0	—	13.4
Median	3,839	1,841	5,619	2	—	19.2

* Per 100,000 population among adults aged 35 and older, age-adjusted to the 1990 U.S. population; rates exclude deaths among infants and burn deaths among persons aged 1–34 years.
† Based on mortality rate.

Comments

Cigarette smoking is the single most preventable cause of premature death in the United States and accounted for more than 400,000 deaths across the nation in 1990. The number of deaths attributable to smoking ranged from a low of 402 in Alaska to 42,574 in California. Utah had the lowest mortality rate (218 per 100,000 population) and the lowest percentage of deaths caused by smoking (13.4%). Neighboring Nevada had the highest mortality rate (478 per 100,000 population) and the highest percentage of deaths from smoking (24%). The estimated average number of smoking-attributable deaths per state was 5,619.

Source

Centers for Disease Control and Prevention. "Surveillance for Smoking-Attributable Mortality and Years of Potential Life Lost, by State—United States, 1990." *Morbidity and Mortality Report* 43, No. SS-1, (1994) pp. 1–8.

Contact

Department of Health and Human Services, Public Health Service, Centers for Disease Control and Prevention, Atlanta, GA 30333. For inquiries about the *Morbidity and Mortality Weekly Report*, call (404) 332-4555. The CDC also maintains a World-Wide Web server at http://www.cdc.gov/.

Relative Risks Attributable to Smoking: 1990

Estimated smoking-attributable mortality per 100,000 people for current and former smokers
compared with nonsmokers, by disease category and gender, 1990

Diseases Among Adults (age 35 yrs. and older)	Males		Females	
	Current Smokers	Former Smokers	Current Smokers	Former Smokers
Neoplasms (tumors)				
Lip, oral cavity, pharynx	27.5	8.8	5.6	2.9
Esophagus	7.6	5.8	10.3	3.2
Pancreas	2.1	1.1	2.3	1.8
Larynx	10.5	5.2	17.8	11.9
Trachea, lung, bronchus	22.4	9.4	11.9	4.7
Cervix uteri	NA	NA	2.1	1.9
Urinary bladder	2.9	1.9	2.6	1.9
Kidney, other urinary	3.0	2.0	1.4	1.2
Cardiovascular Diseases				
Hypertensive diseases	1.9	1.3	1.7	1.2
Ischemic heart disease				
Persons ages 35–64 yrs	2.8	1.8	3.0	1.4
Persons ages 65 and older	1.6	1.3	1.6	1.3
Other heart diseases	1.9	1.3	1.7	1.2
Cerebrovascular Diseases				
Persons ages 35–64 yrs	3.7	1.4	4.8	1.4
Persons ages 65 and older	1.9	1.3	1.5	1.0
Atherosclerosis	4.1	2.3	3.0	1.3
Aortic aneurysm	4.1	2.3	3.0	1.3
Other arterial diseases	4.1	2.3	3.0	1.3
Respiratory Diseases				
Pneumonia and influenza	2.0	1.6	2.2	1.4
Bronchitis and emphysema	9.7	8.8	10.5	7.0
Chronic airway obstruction	9.7	8.8	10.5	7.0
Other respiratory diseases	2.0	1.6	2.2	1.4

NA = not applicable

Comments   The Centers for Disease Control and Prevention's Office on Smoking and Health estimated the number of smoking-related deaths from neoplastic, cardiovascular, and respiratory conditions. These estimates were made using formulas designed to calculate risk. These formulas were based on smoking prevalence and relative risks for certain conditions among current and former smokers.

For example, for every one male *non-smoker* who died of a tumor of the esophagus, there were 5.8 male *former* smokers and 7.6 male *current* smokers who died from the same type of tumor. Not included with this information are statistics regarding burn deaths associ-

ated with smoking, which are estimated from injury surveillance studies to account for 50% of all deaths from burns.

According to this study, current smokers had a much greater risk of dying from several types of neoplasms (tumors) than did non-smokers. For example, for every one male *nonsmoker* who died from lip, oral cavity, and pharynx neoplasms, an estimated 8.8 male *former* smokers and 27.5 male *current* smokers died from that cause.

The adult rates listed show the estimated smoking-attributable mortality per 100,000 population for persons aged 35 and older.

Source   U.S. Department of Health and Human Services. Public Health Service. Centers for Disease Control and Prevention. "Surveillance for Smoking-Attributable Mortality and Years of Potential Life Lost, by State—United States, 1990." *Morbidity and Mortality Report* 43, No. SS-1, (1994) pp. 1–8.

Contact   Department of Health and Human Services, Public Health Service, Centers for Disease Control and Prevention, Atlanta, GA 30333. For inquiries about the *Morbidity and Mortality Weekly Report*, call (404) 332-4555. The CDC also maintains a World-Wide Web server at http://www.cdc.gov/.

Results of Surveys on Prohibiting or Restricting Smoking: 1993

Percentage (and margin of error) of surveyed persons aged 18 and older who were in favor of banning (prohibiting) or restricting smoking in certain public locations. Results of surveys in eight states, 1993.

State	Sample Size	Fast-Food Restaurant		Sit-Down Restaurant		Indoor Malls		Indoor Sporting Events	
		Restrict	Ban	Restrict	Ban	Restrict	Ban	Restrict	Ban
Louisiana	275	47.9 (±6.3)	46.8 (±6.2)	49.1 (±6.3)	44.3 (±6.4)	47.2 (±6.3)	44.0 (±6.1)	34.3 (±5.3)	58.2 (±5.4)
Missouri	254	46.4 (±7.0)	49.0 (±6.9)	55.5 (±6.9)	39.5 (±6.8)	52.0 (±7.5)	39.4 (±7.2)	35.6 (±6.8)	57.8 (±6.6)
New Jersey	261	41.0 (±6.8)	51.0 (±7.0)	49.0 (±7.0)	44.8 (±7.0)	34.1 (±6.3)	46.9 (±7.1)	29.7 (±6.1)	56.4 (±6.9)
Ohio	258	46.8 (±6.9)	50.2 (±6.9)	55.1 (±6.9)	41.2 (±6.8)	56.2 (±6.8)	33.4 (±6.5)	33.6 (±6.4)	55.4 (±6.8)
Oklahoma	252	52.6 (±6.9)	42.5 (±7.0)	54.3 (±6.8)	42.3 (±6.8)	57.5 (±6.8)	35.5 (±7.1)	35.2 (±7.5)	60.8 (±7.7)
South Carolina	371	36.8 (±5.5)	56.8 (±5.6)	46.0 (±5.9)	50.0 (±5.8)	48.4 (±6.2)	45.6 (±6.3)	25.1 (±5.1)	66.9 (±5.2)
Texas	405	41.4 (±5.4)	50.5 (±6.0)	50.0 (±6.2)	45.8 (±5.8)	46.9 (±6.1)	45.3 (±6.0)	34.1 (±5.6)	57.0 (±6.3)
Washington	431	33.1 (±4.9)	63.0 (±5.0)	45.4 (±5.1)	50.6 (±5.1)	39.0 (±5.0)	56.5 (±5.1)	29.1 (±4.6)	66.8 (±4.8)

Comments Public sentiment in recent years has increasingly shown support for regulating tobacco use in public areas. According to the National Cancer Institute's Community Intervention Trial for Smoking Cessation, the most favored locations for restricting smoking include bars, restaurants, bowling alleys, private worksites, and government buildings. Banning was often favored for indoor sports arenas, hospitals, and doctors' offices.

The response categories for this survey include: "allowed in all areas" (do not restrict), "allowed in some areas" (restrict), "not allowed at all" (ban), "don't know," and "refused to answer." Some people believe that such policies infringe upon the rights of smokers, while others believe that smokers may have the freedom to smoke, but do not have the freedom to impose the by-product of that habit (second-hand smoke) upon others. Many cities now have ordinances that prohibit smoking in public areas, office buildings and other areas of commerce where people congregate.

The statistics shown here (percentage and margin of error) only represent the opinions of those surveyed within each state, and do not measure any specific policy or strategic action already taken.

Source U.S. Department of Health and Human Services. Public Health Service. Centers for Disease Control and Prevention. "Attitudes Toward Smoking Policies in Eight States—United States, 1993," Centers for Disease Control and Prevention, *Morbidity and Morality Weekly Report* 43, No. 43, (1994) pp. 786–789.

Contact Department of Health and Human Services, Public Health Service, Centers for Disease Control and Prevention, Atlanta, GA 30333. For inquiries about the *Morbidity and Mortality Weekly Report*, call (404) 332-4555. The CDC also maintains a World-Wide Web server at http://www.cdc.gov/.

Results of Surveys on Effective Strategies to Prevent Teenage Smoking: 1993

Percentage (and margin of error) of surveyed persons aged 18 and older who believed that certain strategies to keep teenagers from smoking would be somewhat or very effective. Results of surveys in eight states, 1993.

State	Sample Size	Ban on School Property	Ban all Cigarette Advertising	Strongly Enforce Laws	Ban all Vending Machines	Increase Price of Cigarettes
Louisiana	275	75.8 (±5.2)	71.9 (±6.1)	85.5 (±4.3)	76.0 (±5.6)	67.0 (±6.4)
Missouri	254	65.3 (±6.2)	54.3 (±7.0)	77.6 (±5.7)	69.3 (±6.2)	62.0 (±6.5)
New Jersey	261	76.4 (±6.2)	70.2 (±6.4)	77.1 (±5.8)	75.6 (±5.7)	62.5 (±6.6)
Ohio	258	72.1 (±6.2)	58.0 (±6.8)	78.8 (±5.9)	75.7 (±5.8)	59.0 (±6.8)
Oklahoma	252	77.8 (±6.2)	70.2 (±6.1)	80.9 (±5.4)	79.3 (±5.5)	55.4 (±6.7)
South Carolina	371	75.8 (±5.1)	60.6 (±5.4)	78.8 (±4.9)	72.9 (±5.4)	58.3 (±5.6)
Texas	405	73.6 (±4.8)	64.9 (±5.9)	77.4 (±4.9)	73.3 (±5.5)	63.0 (±5.8)
Washington	431	72.0 (±4.6)	71.0 (±4.8)	84.3 (±3.7)	78.7 (±4.4)	67.7 (±4.8)

Comments

As part of the American Stop Smoking Intervention Study for Cancer Prevention, the American Cancer Society and the National Cancer Institute surveyed persons in eight states during July–August 1993. The purpose of the survey was to characterize public attitudes regarding strategies that might prevent teenagers from smoking. Each respondent was asked whether they thought the strategies were *not at all* effective, *somewhat* effective, or *very* effective.

Although each of the strategies was believed to be either somewhat or very effective, the strategy with the most support (which ranged from 65.3% in Missouri to 77.8% in Oklahoma) regarded banning all smoking inside and outside school property. Banning all advertising of cigarettes was considered an effective strategy to discourage teenage smoking by a range of 54.3% in Missouri to 71.9% in Louisiana.

High proportions of respondents believed that limiting teenagers' access to tobacco products would be an effective deterrent, including stronger enforcement of laws prohibiting sales to minors, banning all cigarette vending machines, and increasing the price of a pack of cigarettes.

Source

U.S. Department of Health and Human Services. Public Health Service. Centers for Disease Control and Prevention. "Attitudes Toward Smoking Policies in Eight States—United States, 1993," Centers for Disease Control and Prevention, *Morbidity and Morality Weekly Report* 43, No. 43, (1994) pp. 786–789.

Contact

Department of Health and Human Services, Public Health Service, Centers for Disease Control and Prevention, Atlanta, GA 30333. For inquiries about the *Morbidity and Mortality Weekly Report*, call (404) 332-4555. The CDC also maintains a World-Wide Web server at http://www.cdc.gov/.

Glossary

Acapulco Gold. A trade name used to illegally market marijuana, indicating that it was grown in southwestern Mexico.

Acapulco Red. A trade name used to illegally market marijuana, indicating that it was grown in Mexico.

Accuracy. Ability to get the correct (or true) result.

Active client. An individual who: (1) has been admitted to the treatment unit and for whom a treatment plan has been developed; (2) has been seen on scheduled appointment basis at least once during the current year; and (3) has not been discharged from treatment, i.e., continued care is expected to be given this client.

Actual clients in treatment. The actual number of active clients being treated in each type of care/modality and facility location/environment as of the current point prevalence date.

ADAMHA program support funds. Funds received for alcohol or drug abuse treatment from NIAAA, NIDA, or NIMH through direct project grants or contracts (including services and services research).

African Black. A trade name used to illegally market marijuana, indicating that it was grown in Africa.

AIDS. A condition caused by a deadly virus that attacks the body's immune system. The disease is transmitted via body fluids, especially sexual secretions and blood. Intravenous drug users risk getting AIDS from infected needles.

Alcohol-related traffic fatality (ARTF). A death in which any driver, pedestrian, or bicylist had a BAC (blood alcohol concentration/content) of greater that 0.01%. Therefore, the young person killed may or may not have been drinking.

Alcohol. Ethanol, the intoxicating substance in distilled or fermented liquors; a drink containing ethanol.

Alcoholism hospital. An institution that provides 24-hour services for the diagnosis and treatment of alcoholic patients through an organized medical or professional staff and permanent facilities that include inpatient beds, medical and nursing services. Clients residing in this type of hospital setting are receiving services primarily for alcoholism and/or other drugs of abuse.

American Indian/Alaskan Native. A person having origins in any of the original peoples of North America.

Amphetamine. A chemical compound used clinically as a drug for treating hyperactive children or as an appetite suppressant; abused as a central nervous system stimulant.

Analgesic. Any drug used primarily to relieve pain. Examples of analgesics include morphine or opiates.

Analyte. Substance to be measured.

Angel dust. Phencyclidine (PCP); a chemical compound used as a veterinary anesthetic, also illicitly as a psychedelic drug.

Angola Black. A trade name used to illegally market marijuana, indicating that it was grown in Angola.

Atom Bomb. Street name for a combination of heroin and marijuana.

Average see mean.

Aversive techniques. Behavioral approaches to the treatment of drug abusers or alcoholics that include the use of procedures which punish unwanted actions and behaviors.

Backjack. Street term for injecting an opiate.

Backup. Street term for preparing a vein for injection of an opiate.

Bang. Street term for injecting an opiate.

Barbiturates. Any derivative of a synthetic crystalline acid used as a sedative or hypnotic drug, often taken illicitly.

Beam Me Up Scottie. Street name for a combination of PCP and crack.

Bingo. Street term for injecting an opiate.

Black Gold. A trade name used to illegally market marijuana, indicating that it is of high potency.

Black Gungi. A trade name used to illegally market marijuana, indicating that it is grown in India.

Black Hash. Street name for a combination of opium and hashish.

Black, not of hispanic origin. A person having origins in any of the peoples of sub-Saharan Africa or Haiti who does not self-classify as Hispanic.

Blast a joint. Street term for smoking marijuana.

Blast a roach. Street term for smoking marijuana.

Blast a stick. Street term for smoking marijuana.

Blast. Street term for smoking marijuana.

Blood alcohol concentration (BAC). The measure of the amount of alcohol in a person's blood; given in grams per deciliter (g/dL, with 100 grams = one deciliter). The BAC given as a percentage would be equal to the g/dL. In most states, a BAC of between 0.01 and 0.09% is within the legal limit; a BAC of greater than 0.10% would constitute intoxication.

Blow a fix/blow a shot. Street term meaning that an injection of an opiate misses the vein and is wasted in the skin.

Blow coke. Street term for inhaling cocaine.

Blow. Street term for inhaling cocaine.

Blow. Street term for smoking marijuana.

Blue de Hue. A trade name used to illegally market marijuana, indicating that it is grown in Vietnam.

Blue Sky Blond. A trade name used to illegally market marijuana, indicating that it is a high potency variety from Colombia.

Boot. Street term for injecting an opiate.

Brokers. Intermediaries who unite drug traffickers and money launderers and negotiate contracts for money-laundering services.

Burn one. Street term for smoking marijuana.

C & M. Street name for a combination of cocaine and morphine.

Cambodia Red/Cam Red. A trade name used to illegally market marijuana, indicating that it is grown in Cambodia.

Canadian Black. A trade name used to illegally market marijuana, indicating that it is grown in Canada.

Cannabis. Any preparation or chemical derived from the hemp plant, such as marijuana, hashish, or THC, which is used illicitly as a mind-altering drug.

Casas de Cambio. Legitimate or illegitimate currency exchanges in Latin American countries.

Channel swimmer. Street term for a person who injects heroin.

Chase. Street term for smoking cocaine.

Child care services. Services which provide care for minor children of active clients, including supervised activities.

Chipping. Street term for occasionally injecting opiates.

Chromatography. A procedure used to identify substances, such as drugs of abuse in urine, based on separating or extracting the substances, allowing them to move or migrate along a carrier, and then identifying them.

Citrol. A trade name used to illegally market marijuana, indicating that it is a high potency variety grown in Nepal.

Cocaine. A crystalline organic base derived from coca leaves, used illicitly as a euphoria-producing drug which is psychologically addictive.

Colombian Black. A trade name used to illegally market marijuana, indicating that it is grown in Colombia.

Community mental health center (CMCH). Includes services which are provided in a comprehensive manner in order to provide a community service. The services usually provided by CMHCs are outpatient care, inpatient care, partial hospitalization, emergency care and consultation and education.

Concentration. Amount of a drug in a unit of biological fluid, expressed as weight/volume. Urine concentrations are usually expressed either as nanograms per milliliter (ng/ml), as micrograms per milliliter (ug/ml), or milligrams per liter (mg/l). (There are 28,000,000 micrograms in an ounce, and 1,000 nanograms in a microgram.)

Constant dollars. Dollars that have been adjusted for fluctuations in value over time. Converting dollar values to constant dollars enables a researcher to compare the cost of things in 1995 with what they cost in 1952.

Cooker. Street term for injecting an opiate.

Correctional facility. Includes adult or juvenile correctional institutions, reentry and diversion facilities, and prisons.

Cotton Brothers. Street name for a combination of cocaine, heroin, and morphine.

Crack cocaine. A purified form of cocaine in the form of small pieces or chips, usually used illicitly by smoking.

Cranking up. Street term for injecting an opiate.

Criminal justice. Activities which include enforcement, prosecution, and sentencing to apprehend, convict, and punish drug offenders. Although thought of primarily as having supply reduction goals, criminal sanctions also have demand reduction effects by discouraging drug use.

Crisis intervention services. Activities which provide information about the availability of services and/or provide services directly to a person on an outpatient basis when he/she is in a crisis situation. A hotline could provide this service by referring a person for emergency care or to an appropriate treatment unit.

Culican. A trade name used to illegally market marijuana, indicating that it is a high potency variety grown in Mexico.

Current heavy smokers. Those who report smoking more than 25 cigarettes a day.

Current smokers. Persons who report ever having smoked more than 100 cigarettes and are currently smoking.

Cushion. Street term for the vein a drug is injected into; also: channel, gutter, pipe, sewer.

Custodial/domiciliary. Provision of food, shelter, and assistance in routine daily living on a long-term basis for persons with alcohol or other drug-related problems.

Cutoff level. The concentration of a drug in urine, usually in nanograms per milliliter, used to determine whether a specimen is positive or negative for the drug in question.

Daily cigarette smokers. Persons who report smoking more than one cigarette per day during the 30 days before the survey.

Demand reduction. Strategies which attempt to decrease individuals' tendency to use drugs. Efforts provide information and education to potential and casual users about the risks and adverse consequences of drug use, and treatment to drug users who have developed problems from using drugs.

Detection limit. Lowest concentration of a drug that can reliably be detected.

Detoxification (drug). The period of planned withdrawal from drug dependency supported by use of a prescribed medication. If methadone is being used, detoxification cannot exceed 21 days. When methadone detoxification exceeds 21 days, the treatment modality becomes maintenance.

Detoxification (medical). The use of medication under the supervision of medical personnel to systematically reduce or eliminate the effects of alcohol in the body in a hospital or other 24-hour care facility.

Detoxification (social). To systematically reduce or eliminate the effects of alcohol in the body on a drug-free basis, in a specialized nonmedical facility by trained personnel with physician services available when required.

Do a joint. Street term for smoking marijuana.

Do a line. Street term for inhaling cocaine.

Dope smoke. Street term for smoking marijuana.

Drug free. A treatment regimen that does not include any pharmacologic agent or medication as the primary part of the drug treatment including drug detoxification.

Temporary medication may be prescribed in a drug free modality, e.g., short-term use of tranquilizers or clonidine for opiate withdrawal, but the primary treatment method is counseling (individual, group, family, etc.), not pharmacotherapy.

Dusting. Street name for adding PCP, heroin, or another drug to marijuana.

Dynamite. Street name for a combination of cocaine and heroin.

Early intervention services. These services are intended to encourage persons to seek early help for their alcohol and drug problems, provide crisis services, educate the helping professions to recognize persons with substance abuse problems and to offer appropriate services, and the like.

Emergency gun. Street term for an instrument other than a syringe used to inject drugs.

Environment. The physical setting and circumstances in which the drug abuse or alcoholism client receives treatment.

Estimate. A rough or approximate calculation used to find a value when there is incomplete data to ascertain the actual value.

False negative. An erroneous result that indicates the absence of a drug that is present.

False positive. An erroneous result that indicates the presence of a drug that is not present.

Family counseling/therapy services. Services which are provided during the same session to members of a family/collateral group.

Fatality. A death caused by an accident, a drug overdose, etc.

Fetal alcohol syndrome (FAS). A birth defect characterized by a variety of physical and behavioral traits that result from maternal alcohol consumption during pregnancy.

Fire it up. Street term for smoking marijuana.

Fix. Street term for injecting an opiate.

Flag. Street term for the appearance of blood in a vein into which a drug has been injected.

Former smokers. Persons who report ever having smoked more than 100 cigarettes but are not currently smoking.

Freebasing. Street term for smoking cocaine.

Frisco Special. Street name for a combination of cocaine, heroin, and LSD.

Frisco Speedball. Street name for a combination of cocaine, heroin, and LSD.

Fuel. Street name for a combination of marijuana and insecticides.

Fuete. Street term for hypodermic needle; also: gaffus, glass, glass gun, hype stick.

Geeze. Street term for inhaling cocaine.

Geezer. Street term for injecting an opiate.

General hospital, including veteran's administration (VA) hospitals. Nonspecialized acute care hospitals where the average length of stay for a patient is usually less than 30 days. A VA hospital is a hospital which operates under the auspices of the Veteran's Administration.

Get a gage up. Street term for smoking marijuana.

Get off. Street term for injecting an opiate.

Ghost busting. Street term for smoking cocaine.

Goofball. Street name for a combination of cocaine and heroin.

Group counseling/therapy services. Services which are provided to a group of clients by unit staff members. This would include but not be limited to psychotherapy, insight therapy, reality therapy, transactional analysis, and the various types of expressive groups.

Halfway house/recovery home. A community-based, peer group oriented, residential facility that provides food, shelter, and supportive services (including vocational, recreational, social services) in a supportive non-drug use, non-drinking environment for the ambulatory and mentally competent recovering substance abuser who may be reentering the work force. It also provides or arranges for provision of appropriate treatment services.

Hallucinogen. A drug or any substance that produces hallucinations.

Hawaiian. A trade name used to illegally market marijuana, indicating that it is a variety of very high potency grown in Hawaii.

Herb and Al. Street name for combining marijuana and alcohol.

Heroin. A highly addictive narcotic drug, similar to, but more potent than, morphine. Used for its effect of extreme euphoria. Illegal for medical use in the United States.

Hispanic. A person of Cuban, Mexican, Puerto Rican, and all other Spanish cultures and origins, regardless of race (includes Central and South America and Spain).

Hit the hay. Street term for smoking marijuana.

Hit the main line. Street term for injecting an opiate.

Hit. Street term for smoking marijuana.

Hitch up the reindeers. Street term for inhaling cocaine.

HIV. Human immunodeficiency virus; one of a group of retroviruses that destroy the human immune system; producing the disease known as AIDS.

Hospital, inpatient. An institution that provides 24-hour services for the diagnosis and treatment of patients through an organized medical or professional staff and permanent licensed medical/psychiatric facilities that include inpatient beds, medical, and nursing services. Patients residing in hospital settings should be receiving services primarily for alcoholism and/or other drugs of abuse.

Hot load/hot shot. Street term for a lethal injection of an opiate.

Hotline. A telephone service that provides information and referral and immediate counseling, frequently in a crisis situation.

Illicit drug. A drug used unlawfully, usually for mind-altering purposes.

Immunoassay. A procedure used to identify substances, such as drugs of abuse in urine, based on the competition between tagged and untagged antigen to combine with antibodies. The uncombined, tagged antigen is an indicator of the drug present in the urine specimen.

Indian Boy. A trade name used to illegally market marijuana, indicating that it is grown in India.

Indian Hay. A trade name used to illegally market marijuana from an Indian hemp plant.

Indica. A trade name used to illegally market marijuana, indicating that it is one of the varieties of cannabis found in hot climates, often growing to 3.5 to 4 feet tall.

Individual counseling/therapy services. Services which are provided to a client on a one-to-one basis.

Interdiction. The interference with the movement of illegal drugs from the source of supply to the point of sale. Methods of interdiction include destruction of crops and seizure of drugs in transport.

Interfering substances. Substances other than the analyte that give a similar analytical response or alter the analytical result.

Jolt. Street term for injecting an opiate.

Joy pop. Street term for injecting an opiate.

Jurisdiction. The sphere of authority of an administrative agency. For example, a sheriff has jurisdiction over the county in which he or she resides.

Kentucky Blue. A trade name used to illegally market marijuana, indicating that it is grown in Kentucky.

Licit drug. A legal drug; a prescription medication.

Local government funds. Provided by local government (city, county, etc.) to provide drug abuse or alcoholism treatment services.

Lock up. This term refers to individuals who have been arrested and locked up in a jail awaiting further legal procedures. A person who has been locked up may subsequently be released without being charged with a crime, or released pending a trial on crimes they are accused of committing. Consequently, because a person has been locked up does not mean he or she is guilty of the crime for which they are being held.

LSD. Lysergic acid diethylamide; an organic compound that causes psychotic symptoms, used illicitly to produce a psychedelic effect.

Main line. Street term for injecting an opiate.

Maintenance. The continued administering of methadone and other approved pharmacological adjuncts at relatively stable dosage levels as an oral substitute for opiates among opiate dependent clients. Maintenance may be provided in conjunction with appropriate social and medical services. This category also includes those clients who are being withdrawn from maintenance treatment.

Mandatory. Something that is required and not voluntary. In some industries, drug testing is mandatory. In other words, if an employee refuses to submit to a drug test, he or she will lose their job.

Manhattan Silver. A trade name used to illegally market marijuana, indicating that it is from Manhattan, New York.

Marijuana. The dried leaves and flowers of the hemp plant, usually illicitly smoked as a cigarette for its intoxicating effect.

Maui Wauie. A trade name used to illegally market marijuana, indicating that it is grown in Hawaii.

Mean. A single number that broadly describes an entire set of numbers. A mean (commonly called an "average") is calculated by adding the values of all the cases and dividing by the total number of cases. For the set of values [2, 3, 3, 5, 6, 6, 10] the mean is 7.

Median. The quantity or value of the case within a series of cases where one-half of all cases have values greater than the case itself and the other one-half of the cases have values less than the case itself. For the set of values [2, 3, 3, 5, 6, 6, 10] the median is 5.

Mental/psychiatric hospital. A medical facility which offers short-term intensive inpatient treatment and prolonged inpatient treatment to persons suffering from a variety of mental or psychiatric disorders, including alcohol and drug-related disorders. Such facilities can be public or private.

Metabolite. A compound produced from chemical changes of a drug in the body.

Methadone treatment. Refers to methadone maintenance or detoxification. Methadone maintenance is the continued administering of methadone, in conjunction with provision of appropriate social and medical services, at relatively stable dosage levels for 21 days or more. Methadone is used as an oral substitute for opiates during the rehabilitative phase of treatment. This category also includes those clients who are being withdrawn from maintenance treatment.

Methadone. A synthetic drug used as a substitute narcotic to treat heroin addiction or relieve pain; abused as an addictive and narcotic drug in itself.

Methamphetamine. A form of amphetamine, a chemical compound used clinically as a drug for treating hyperactive children or as an appetite suppressant; abused as a central nervous system stimulant.

Mexican Brown. A trade name used to illegally market marijuana, indicating that it is grown in Mexico.

Mode. The most frequently occurring member of a set of numbers. For the set of values [2, 3, 3, 5, 6, 6, 10] there are two modes, 3 and 6, since both values occur most often.

Morphine. The principal narcotic organic base of opium, used clinically to relieve pain or as a sedative; abused as an addictive narcotic.

Mow the grass. Street term for smoking marijuana.

Mules. People who actually smuggle drugs or drug money by carrying it on their person.

Never smokers. Persons who report that they have smoked less than 100 cigarettes.

Offshore banks. Financial institutions in foreign countries that usually have bank secrecy laws and are often tax havens.

Opiate. A derivative of opium, a broad term for a narcotic.

Opium. An addictive narcotic drug derived from the opium poppy.

Outpatient facility. An establishment or a distinct part of an establishment, which is primarily engaged in providing drug abuse or alcoholism services for persons who reside elsewhere. This term is included on page 1 in Item C, Unit's Location and on the drug matrix on Page 2 as an environment.

Outpatient. Treatment/recovery/aftercare, or rehabilitation services provided by a facility where the client does not reside in a treatment facility. The client receives drug abuse or alcoholism treatment services with or without medication, including counseling and supportive services. Daycare is included in this category. This is also known as non-residential services in the alcoholism field.

Outreach services. Outreach activities involve efforts in the community for early case-finding and early intervention services to drug and alcohol abusers. These services would also include efforts to educate various groups about drug and alcohol abuse.

Pakistani Black. A trade name used to illegally market marijuana, indicating that it is grown in Pakistan.

Panama Gold A trade name used to illegally market marijuana, indicating that it is grown in Panama.

Panama Red. A trade name used to illegally market marijuana, indicating that it is grown in Panama.

PCP. Phencyclidine; a chemical compound used as a veterinary anesthetic, also illicitly as a psychedelic drug. Also known as angel dust.

Physical examination. A medical examination by (or supervised by) a physician or other health professional to determine the status of an individual's health.

Pigeons. Intermediaries who steer traffickers to money-launderers for a set price.

Poke. Street term for smoking marijuana.

Pop. Street term for inhaling cocaine.

Precision. Ability to get the same result in repeated measurements.

Presumed positive. A specimen identified at or above the screening test threshold but not yet subjected to confirmation testing.

Prevention. Educational efforts to inform potential users about the health, legal, and other risks associated with drug use. Their goal is to limit the number of new drug users and dissuade casual users from continuing drug use as part of a demand reduction strategy.

Prevention/education. Those activities that are intended to reduce or minimize the incidence of new drug abuse or alcoholism problems and the negative consequences of the use of alcohol and/or licit or illicit drugs. Available services may vary widely but are generally associated with information, education, alternatives, and primary and early intervention activities, and may also encompass services such as literature distribution, media campaigns, clearinghouse activities, speaker's bureau, and school or peer group situations. These services may be directed at any segment of the population.

Prohibition. The ban on the distribution, possession, and use of special substances made illegal by legislative or administrative order and the application of criminal penalties to violators.

Public inebriates. Individuals who are habitually intoxicated in public places.

Public welfare Medical or social service benefits or payments made available through local general assistance or general relief programs, including food stamps.

Puff the dragon. Street term for smoking marijuana.

Random sample. A sampling from some population where each entry has an equal chance of being drawn. Random sampling is used to obtain significant statistics about groups too large to sample individually.

Recovery. A process to develop and sustain an abstinent life-style within a helping context of mutual aid from drug free peers and adherence to principles of behavior that promote sobriety.

Regulation. Control over the distribution, possession, and use of specified substances. Regulations specify the circumstances under which substances can be legally distributed and used. Prescription medications and alcohol are the substances most commonly regulated in the U.S.

Rehabilitation/recovery. An approach which provides a planned program of professionally directed evaluation, care, and treatment for the restoration of functioning for persons impaired by drug abuse or alcoholism.

Representative sample. A sample so large and average in composition that it can be said to accurately represent the larger group from which it was drawn.

Research services. Activities performed by unit staff to systematically collect and/or analyze empirical data based on the scientific model of developing knowledge.

Residential facility. A live-in setting where nonmedical rehabilitative drug abuse and/or alcoholism services are available to residents, e.g., foster homes, group homes, or boarding houses.

Residential. Assessment, diagnosis, care, and treatment to clients who reside in a nonmedical treatment facility (other than a prison or hospital) that provides residential support, ambulatory care during the treatment and rehabilitation process including counseling, group therapy and other health-related services. Residential facilities include quarterway house, halfway house/recovery homes, group homes and therapeutic communities.

Ruderalis. A trade name used to illegally market marijuana, indicating that it is one of the varieties found in Russia, growing 1 to 2.5 feet tall.

Sativa. A trade name used to illegally market marijuana, indicating that it is one of the varieties found in cool, damp climates, often growing up to 18 feet tall.

Self-help groups. Independent support groups or fellowships organized by and for drug abusers, alcoholics or their collaterals to help members achieve and maintain abstinence from and/or cope with the effects of licit or illicit drugs and alcohol. Examples are Alcoholics Anonymous, Narcotics Anonymous, Women for Sobriety, Al Anon or other non-professionally led groups such as Al Anon-Adult Children of Alcoholics.

Sensitivity. The ability of a procedure to detect minute amounts of substances. A highly sensitive procedure will rarely fail to detect a substance if it is present; thus, few false negative results will occur.

Shell corporations. Corporations established to hide or launder money from illegal drug operations that do not actually engage in the business they are incorporated to perform.

Shoot/shoot up. Street term for injecting an opiate.

Skin popping. Street term for injecting an opiate.

Slam. Street term for injecting an opiate.

Smokeless tobacco. A pulverized form of tobacco which is chewed or held between the cheek and gums.

Smurfing. Making numerous currency transactions usually converting cash into money orders or cashiers checks that are each under the reporting requirement of $10,000 in order to avoid reporting.

Smurfs. People who make the currency transactions in smurfing.

Sniff. Street term for inhaling cocaine.

Snort. Street term for inhaling cocaine. Toot. Street term for inhaling cocaine.

Space Cadet. Street name for a combination of PCP and crack.

Specialized hospital. Includes hospitals that emphasize the diagnosis and treatment of particular disorders, e.g., psychiatric, children, epilepsy, maternity, orthopedics, etc.

Specificity. The ability of a procedure to differentiate between chemically similar substances. A highly specific procedure is rarely positive for a given drug if the substance is truly absent, thus few false positive results will occur.

Speedball. Street name for a combination of cocaine and heroin.

Spike. Street term for injecting an opiate.

Straws. People who stand in for actual owners of businesses and shell corporations in order to hide ownership.

Structuring. Arranging currency deposits in order to avoid reporting requirements.

Substance abuse. Use of a substance, such as alcohol or drugs, to excess or without medical necessity.

Substance. A term for drugs or alcoholic beverages which are usually considered harmful and are regulated by laws.

Supply reduction. Strategies which focus diplomatic, law enforcement, military, and other resources on eliminating or reducing the supply of drugs. Efforts focus on foreign countries, smuggling routes outside the country, border interdiction, and distribution within the U.S.

Taxation. Requires those who produce, distribute, or possess drugs to pay a fee based on the volume or value of the drugs. Failure to pay subjects violators to penalties for this violation, not for the drug activities themselves.

Tea party. Street term for smoking marijuana.

Teen suicide prevention services. Services for youth, family members, and peers designed to educate, prevent, or intervene in teen suicidal behavior.

Testing. Procedures that test individuals for the presence of drugs. Testing is a tool in drug control that is used for safety and monitoring purposes and as an adjunct to therapeutic interventions. It is in widespread use for employees in certain jobs such as those in the transportation industry and criminal justice agencies. New arrestees and convicted offenders may be tested. Individuals in treatment are often tested to monitor their progress and provide them an incentive to remain drug free.

Tex-Mex. A trade name used to illegally market marijuana, indicating that it is grown in the southwestern U.S.

Texas Pot. A trade name used to illegally market marijuana, indicating that it is grown in Texas.

Texas Tea. A trade name used to illegally market marijuana, indicating that it is grown in Texas.

THC. Tetrahydrocannabinol; the chemical derived from the hemp plant that is the main intoxicant in marijuana.

Tobacco. The leaves of the cultivated tobacco plant, a member of the nightshade family, used for smoking as cigarettes or for chewing, as smokeless tobacco.

Toke up. Street term for smoking marijuana.

Toke. Street term for smoking marijuana.

Tragic Magic. Street name for a combination of PCP and crack.

Tranquilizers. Any drug that produces a calming effect without inducing sleep. Tranquilizers are used to relieve anxiety and achieve peace of mind. Although tranquilizers are useful and important drugs prescribed by doctors, they are also prone to substance abuse.

Treatment (not methadone). Formal organized services for persons who have abused alcohol and/or other drugs. These services are designed to alter specific physical, mental, or social functions of persons receiving care by reducing disability or discomfort, and ameliorate the signs or symptoms caused by alcohol and/or drug abuse. This is also referred to as recovery services in some States.

Treatment unit. A facility having: (1) a formal structured arrangement for alcohol or drug abuse treatment or recovery using alcohol or drug-specified personnel; and (2) a designated portion of the facility (or resources) for treatment services; and (3) an allocated budget for such treatment services. A treatment unit must directly provide services to clients at the facility's location. The unit usually offers some form of initial evaluation or diagnosis of its clients and, thereafter, may include a wide range of different services, such as counseling, job placement, or other rehabilitation services. This is also referred to as a recovery unit in some States.

Treatment. Therapeutic interventions that focus on individuals whose drug use has caused medical, psychological, economic, and social problems for them. The interventions may include medication, counseling, and other support services delivered in an inpatient setting or on an outpatient basis. These are demand reduction activities to eliminate or reduce individuals' drug use.

Up against the stem. Street term meaning addicted to smoking marijuana.

User accountability. A policy emphasizing that all users of illegal substances, regardless of the type of drug they use or the frequency of that use, are violating criminal laws and should be subject to penalties. It is closely associated with zero tolerance.

Wac. Street name for a combination of PCP and marijuana.

White, not of hispanic origin. A Caucasian person having origins in any of the people of Europe (includes Portugal), North Africa, or the Middle East.

Wire transfers. Electronic communication of funds between financial institutions both within the U.S. and abroad.

Young drivers involved in fatal crashes. Drivers aged 15 to 20 involved in a crash that resulted in a fatality. these drivers may have been fatally injured or survived the crash, or the fatality may have been a youth or adult.

Young drivers killed. Drivers aged 15 to 20 who were killed in a motor vehicle crash.

Youth fatalities (alcohol-related). Those who died in motor vehicle crashes (drivers, passengers, or non-occupant) who were 15 to 20 years old.

Zacatecas Purple. A trade name used to illegally market marijuana, indicating that it is grown in Mexico.

Zero tolerance. A policy that holds that drug distributors, buyers, and users should be held fully accountable for their offenses under the law.

Zoom. Street name for a combination of PCP and marijuana.

Index

A

Accidents
    drug use and emergency room visits: 167
Adult education
    alcohol use demographics (1991): 8, 9
ADAMHA *see* Alcohol, Drug Abuse, and Mental Health Administration
Afghanistan
    hashish production (1988–93): 64, 65
    opium production (1988–93): 60
    world opium supply: 57, 61
Age
    adolescent drinking and smoking (1992): 16, 17
    alcohol consumption (1974–91): 6, 7
    alcohol use demographics (1991): 8, 9
    alcohol-related youth fatalities (1985–93): 28, 29
    arrests for drunkenness (1993): 42, 43
    blood alcohol concentrations (BACs) of fatally injured drivers (1993): 22, 23
    cigarette smoking by high school seniors (1975–94): 188, 189
    cigarette smoking by youths aged 12–21 (1992): 190, 191
    convicted drug felons: 114, 115
    cost of smoking-related sickness (1987): 198, 199
    drinking and other unhealthy behaviors in adolescents (1992): 14, 15
    drug use sampling of past month (1992): 84, 85
    DUI arrests (1993) of persons under 18 years: 36
    liquor use and role in violent behavior (1993–94): 87
    lives saved by drinking age laws (1985–93): 28, 29
    marijuana use and role in violent behavior (1993–94): 86, 87
    past month drug use (18–25 year olds) (1974–91): 88, 89
    problems associated with alcohol use (1991): 4, 5
    reasons for cigarette use (1993): 194, 195
    reported nicotine withdrawal symptoms (1993): 196, 197
    steroid use by high school seniors (1989–94): 90, 91
    teenagers' use of smokeless tobacco (1986–94): 192, 193

total arrests for DUI (1993): 38, 39
    youth crash fatalities and alcohol (1982–93): 32–35
Age groups
    cigarette smokers (1992): 185
    relative risks attributable to smoking (1990): 204
Aggravated assault
    felony convictions in state courts (1992): 118
AIDS
    drug use transmission: 165
Air Force: 93
    drug use (1992): 92, 93
Air interdiction: 135
Aircraft
    seizure by the DEA (1992): 146
Alabama
    cannabis eradication efforts (1990): 142
    cigarette smokers aged 35 and over (1990): 182
    deaths attributed to smoking (1990): 202
    motor vehicle crash fatalities (1993): 20
    potential years of life lost by cigarette smoking (1990): 200
Alaska
    cannabis eradication efforts (1990): 142
    cigarette smokers aged 35 and over (1990): 182
    deaths attributed to smoking (1990): 202, 203
    drug abuse surveys: 7
    motor vehicle crash fatalities (1993): 20
    potential years of life lost by cigarette smoking (1990): 200
Alcohol
    motor vehicle crash fatalities by state (1993): 21
    adolescent use of (1992): 16, 17, 191
    alcohol-related arrests (1972–93): 40, 41
    alcohol-related youth fatalities (1985–93): 28, 29
    arrests for drunkenness (1993): 42, 43
    blood alcohol concentrations (BACs) of fatally injured drivers (1993): 22, 23
    consumption by age group (1974–91): 6, 7
    deaths in the workplace (1992): 96, 97
    deaths induced (1979–92): 50, 51
    demographic characteristics of users (1991): 8
    drunkenness arrests in the U.S. (1993) by population group: 44, 45

DUI arrests (1993): 36, 37
fatal traffic injuries involving (1983–93): 18, 19
fatal workplace injuries (1992): 46, 47
fatalities in alcohol-related traffic accidents (1982–91): 24, 25
fatally injured drunk drivers (1980–93): 30, 31
fetal alcohol syndrome rates (1979–93): 48, 49
involvement in automobile crashes (1988–91): 26, 27
lives saved by drinking age laws (1985–93): 28, 29
motor vehicle crash fatalities by state (1993): 20
past month use (1974–91): 10, 11
problems with frequency of use (1991): 2, 3
problems with use by age groups (1991): 4, 5
total arrests: 38, 39
use by adolescents (1992): 14, 15
use by high school seniors (1982–93): 12, 13
use of as transition: 69
youth crash fatalities (1982–93): 32–35
Alcohol and Drug Abuse Education Act amendments: 54
Alcohol dependence syndrome: 51
Alcohol impaired: 47
Alcohol poisoning: 51
Alcohol prohibition: 54
Alcohol psychoses: 51
Alcohol treatment
census of clients in (1980–92): 172, 173
Alcohol use
among high school seniors (1991–94): 77
Alcohol, Drug Abuse, and Mental Health Administration (ADAMHA): 177
Alcoholic cardiomyopathy: 51
Alcoholic gastritis: 51
Alcoholic polyneuropathy: 51
Alcohol-related arrests and DUI (1972–93): 40, 41
Alcohol-related fatality
definition: 35
Alcohol-related offenses
definition: 41
American Cancer Society: 209
American Indian/Alaskan Natives
prevalence of smoking: 185
American Stop Smoking Intervention Study for Cancer Prevention: 209
Amphetamines: 82
DEA ranking schedule: 80
deaths in the workplace (1992): 96
drug laboratory seizures (1975–91): 136
effects of: 78
U.S. expenditures on (1988–93): 153
use by U.S. military personnel (1992): 92

use during crimes (1990): 104, 105
Amyl nitrates
use among high school seniors (1991–94): 76, 77
Anabolic steroids: 91
DEA ranking schedule: 80
use by high school seniors (1989–94): 90, 91
use by U.S. military personnel: 92, 93
Analgesics
mind-altering effects of: 79
use by U.S. military personnel: 92, 93
Angola
marijuana production (1988–93): 63
Antidepressants
deaths in the workplace (1992): 96
Anti-Drug Abuse Act: 55, 125, 131
Any drug
use by U.S. military personnel (1992): 92
Any drug except marijuana
use by U.S. military personnel (1992): 92
Any illicit drug
use among high school seniors (1991–94): 76
Aortic aneurysm
relative risks attributable to smoking (1990): 204
Arizona
cannabis eradication efforts (1990): 142
cigarette smokers aged 35 and over (1990): 182
deaths attributed to smoking (1990): 202
motor vehicle crash fatalities (1993): 20
potential years of life lost by cigarette smoking (1990): 200
Arkansas
cannabis eradication efforts (1990): 142
cigarette smokers aged 35 and over (1990): 182
deaths attributed to smoking (1990): 202
motor vehicle crash fatalities (1993): 20
potential years of life lost by cigarette smoking (1990): 200
Army
drug use (1992): 92, 93
Arrests
drug-related (1988–93): 102
Arson
drug use during (1990): 105
Arterial diseases
relative risks attributable to smoking (1990): 204
Asia
drug smuggling to U.S.: 67
Asian/Pacific Islanders
prevalence of smoking: 185
Assault
drug use during (1990): 104, 105

costs to society from drug use: 164
drug use and emergency room visits: 167
Asset forfeiture laws: 147
Asset seizure by the DEA: 146–148
Atherosclerosis
relative risks attributable to smoking (1990): 204

B

BAC *see* Blood alcohol concentration
Barbiturates: 82
deaths in the workplace (1992): 96
U.S. expenditures on (1988–93): 153
use among high school seniors (1991–94): 76, 77
use by U.S. military personnel (1992): 92
use during crimes (1990): 104, 105
Baseline year: 29
BDMP *see* Birth Defects Monitoring Program
Belize
marijuana production (1988–93): 62
marijuana supplier: 57
Benzedrine®
DEA ranking schedule: 80
Benzodiazepine: 82, 83
use during crimes (1990): 104, 105
Birth Defects Monitoring Program (BDMP): 49
Blackmail disputes
drug use during (1990): 105
Blood alcohol concentration (BAC): 19, 21, 24, 25, 46, 47
of fatally injured drivers (1993): 22
Boggs Act: 54
Bolivia
cocaine production (1992, 1993): 58
wholesale cocaine prices (1991): 162
Border policing
as a supply reduction tactic: 125
Bronchial tumors
relative risks attributable to smoking (1990): 204
Bronchitis
relative risks attributable to smoking (1990): 204
Buds (marijuana)
THC content of seized (1975–90): 100, 101
Bureau of Alcohol, Tobacco, and Firearms: 149
Bureau of Indian Affairs: 141
Bureau of Justice Statistics: 103
Bureau of Labor Statistics: 95, 97
Bureau of Labor Statistics' Census of Fatal
Occupational Injuries *see* Census of Fatal
Occupational Injuries(CFOI)

Bureau of Land Management: 141
Burglaries
costs to society from drug use: 164
Burglary
drug use during (1990): 104, 105
felony convictions in state courts (1992): 118
Burma
coca leaf and opium supplier: 57
opium production (1988–93): 60
world opium supply: 57, 61
Burn deaths
relative risks attributable to smoking (1990): 205
Butyl nitrates
use among high school seniors (1991–94): 76, 77

C

California
cannabis eradication efforts (1990): 142
cigarette smokers aged 35 and over (1990): 182, 183
deaths attributed to smoking (1990): 202, 203
motor vehicle crash fatalities (1993): 20
potential years of life lost by cigarette smoking (1990): 200
Cambodia
marijuana production (1988–93): 63
Canada
drug smuggling to U.S.: 67
marijuana production (1988–93): 63
Cannabis: 101
destruction in the states (1982–90): 140
eradication efforts (1990): 142, 143
federal seizures of (1989–93): 132, 133
hashish production: 64, 65
Cardiovascular diseases
relative risks attributable to smoking (1990): 204, 205
CDC *see* Centers for Disease Control and Prevention
Census of Fatal Occupational Injuries (CFOI),
Bureau of Labor Statistics : 47, 97
Centers for Disease Control and Prevention (CDC): 51, 185, 195, 197, 199, 205
U.S. mortality (death) statistics: 169
Central America
drug smuggling to U.S.: 67
Cerebrovascular diseases
relative risks attributable to smoking (1990): 204
Cervix uteri, tumors of
relative risks attributable to smoking (1990): 204
CFOI *see* Census of Fatal Occupational Injuries
Chewing tobacco *see* Tobacco (smokeless)

Chicago, IL
cocaine, retail price per gram (1986–91): 158
drug use by arrested persons (1991): 83
Chronic airway obstruction
relative risks attributable to smoking (1990): 204
Chronic liver disease: 51
Chronic obstructive pulmonary disease
women cigarette smokers and: 187
Cigarette smokers
high school seniors (1975–94): 188, 189
race, education, age, and income (1992): 184, 185
youths aged 12–21 (1992): 190, 191
women aged 18–44 (1987–92): 186, 187
Cigarette smoking
deaths attributed to (1990): 202, 203
potential years of life lost (1990): 200, 201
prevalence of selected reasons for use (1993): 194, 195
relative risks attributable to (1990): 204
results of surveys on effective strategies to prevent
teenage smoking (1993): 208, 209
surveys on prohibition or restriction of (1993): 206,
207
Cigarette smoking-related sickness
cost of medical care (1987): 198, 199
Cigarettes
per capita yearly consumption (1900–94): 180, 181
smokers aged 35 and over by state (1990): 182, 183
Cirrhosis: 51
Coca leaf
world production of (1987–91): 56
Cocaine: 83–89
adolescent use: 191
annual consumption (1972–92): 74, 75
DEA ranking schedule: 80
deaths in the workplace (1992): 96, 97
effects of: 78
emergency room episodes (1988–93): 166, 167
estimated number of users (1988–93): 72, 73
federal seizures of (1989–93): 132, 133
individuals reporting drug use (1993): 68, 69
international drug seizures (1989–93): 138, 139
land and marine seizures (1976–92): 134, 135
mind-altering effects of: 79
processing and refining: 57
retail price per gram by region (1986–91): 158
retail prices per gram (1988–93): 154, 155
smuggling, by mode of transportation (1986): 66, 67
trends of use (1979–93): 70, 71
U.S. expenditures on (1988–93): 152, 153
use among high school seniors (1991–94): 76
use by adolescents (1992): 14
use by U.S. military personnel (1992): 92
use during crimes (1990): 104, 105
use during past month (1974–91): 88
wholesale prices for (1991): 162, 163
worldwide production (1992, 1993): 59
Cocaine, powdered
state and local narcotics enforcement (1990): 144, 145
Codeine
DEA ranking schedule: 80
deaths in the workplace (1992): 96
Codeine/aspirin
DEA ranking schedule: 80
Codeine/Tylenol®
DEA ranking schedule: 80
College students
drug abuse surveys: 7
Colombia
cocaine production (1992, 1993): 58
marijuana production (1988–93): 62, 63
marijuana supplier: 57
opium production (1988–93): 60
wholesale cocaine prices (1991): 162
wholesale prices for marijuana (1991): 160, 161
Colorado
cannabis eradication efforts (1990): 142
cigarette smokers aged 35 and over (1990): 182
deaths attributed to smoking (1990): 202
motor vehicle crash fatalities (1993): 20
potential years of life lost by cigarette smoking (1990):
200
Commercial grade marijuana
THC content of seized (1975–90): 100
Communications and public utilities
drug testing programs (1989): 94
Community Mental Health Centers Act: 54
Comprehensive Crime Control Act: 55
Comprehensive Drug Abuse and Prevention Act,
1984: 149
Confidence interval
cigarette smoking: 185
Connecticut
cannabis eradication efforts (1990): 143
cigarette smokers aged 35 and over (1990): 182
deaths attributed to smoking (1990): 202
motor vehicle crash fatalities (1993): 20
potential years of life lost by cigarette smoking (1990):
200
Construction
drug testing programs (1989): 94
Continuing criminal enterprise
federal drug convictions (1985–92): 120
Controlled Substances Act: 54, 81

Conveyances
  seizure by the DEA (1992): 146
Corrections
  state and local spending (1991): 126
Crack cocaine
  effects of: 78
  individuals reporting drug use (1993): 69
  state and local narcotics enforcement (1990): 144
  use among high school seniors (1991–94): 76
  use during past month (1974–91): 88
Crash fatalities
  definition: 35
Crime Control Act: 55
Crimes
  drug use during (1990): 104, 105
Criminal Justice Statistics Association: 131
Criminal justice system, U.S.
  handling of drug cases (1992): 108
Criminal organizations
  asset forfeiture funds from seizures (1986–90): 148
Crystal methamphetamine
  use among high school seniors (1991–94): 76
Currency
  seizure by the DEA (1992): 146
Current smoker
  definition of: 191
Customs Department: 54
Customs Forfeiture Fund: 149

D

Dallas, TX
  drug use by arrested persons (1991): 82
Darvon®
  DEA ranking schedule: 80
DAWN see Drug Abuse Warning Network
DEA see Drug Enforcement Administration
Deaths see Mortality rate: 96
Delaware
  cannabis eradication efforts (1990): 143
  cigarette smokers aged 35 and over (1990): 182
  deaths attributed to smoking (1990): 202
  motor vehicle crash fatalities (1993): 20
  potential years of life lost by cigarette smoking (1990):
    200
Demand reduction tactics: 125
Demerol®
  DEA ranking schedule: 80
Demographics: 114
  alcohol use (1991): 8, 9

cigarette smokers (1992): 185
drunkenness arrests in the U.S. (1993): 44, 45
DUI arrests (1993): 36
Denver, CO
  drug use by arrested persons (1991): 82
Department of Defense see U.S. Department of
  Justice
Department of Defense Authorization Act see U.S.
  Department of Defense
Department of Health and Human Services see U.S.
  Department of Health and Human Services
Department of Justice see U.S. Department of Justice
Department of Justice Asset Forfeiture Fund see U.S.
  Department of Justice
Department of Transportation see U.S. Department of
  Transportation
  drug testing of employees: 95
Department of Veterans Affairs see U.S. Department
  of Veterans Affairs
Depressants: 54
  state and local narcotics enforcement (1990): 144
Designer drugs
  DEA ranking schedule: 80
  state and local narcotics enforcement (1990): 144
  use by U.S. military personnel (1992): 92
Detox
  emergency room episodes (1993): 170, 171
  estimated costs of: 177
Detroit, MI
  drug use by arrested persons (1991): 82
Dexedrine®
  DEA ranking schedule: 80
Diazepam
  DEA ranking schedule: 80
Disorderly conduct: 40, 41
District of Columbia
  cigarette smokers aged 35 and over (1990): 182
  deaths attributed to smoking (1990): 202
  fatal occupational injuries: 47
  motor vehicle crash fatalities (1993): 20
  potential years of life lost by cigarette smoking (1990):
    200
Dogs
  used to detect smuggling: 135
Domestic Cannabis Eradication/Suppression
  Program: 140, 141, 143
Domestic violence
  alcohol abuse and: 5
Driving under the influence (DUI)
  alcohol abuse and: 5

alcohol-related arrests (1972–93): 40, 41
arrests: 37
arrests by selected characteristics (1993): 36
definition and description: 39
ratios: 37
total arrests (1993): 38, 39
Drug Abuse Control amendments: 54
Drug Abuse Education Act: 54
Drug Abuse Office and Treatment Act: 54
Drug Abuse Prevention Treatment and Rehabilitation
amendments: 54
Drug abuse treatment
estimated costs of: 176
emergency room episodes (1993): 171
Drug Abuse Warning Network (DAWN): 171
Drug cases
handling of (1992): 108, 109
Drug control policies
federal spending: 125
punishment for drug trafficking: 119
Drug control spending
federal (1982–93) by category: 122–125
state and local (1991): 126, 127
Drug convictions
federal (1985–92): 120, 121
Drug distribution
federal drug convictions (1985–92): 120, 121
Drug education
as a demand reduction tactic: 125
state and local spending (1991): 126
Drug enforcement
illegal drug laboratory seizures (1975–91): 137
local and state law enforcement agencies (1990): 128,
129
multiagency task forces: 130, 131
Drug Enforcement Administration (DEA): 81, 125,
141, 143, 146, 149
assessment of risk of dependence: 79
drug laboratory seizures (1975–91): 136
economic strategy: 155
ranking specific drugs: 80
Drug episodes: 166
Drug felons
demographic characteristics of (1992): 114, 115
Drug felony sentences
average lengths of (1992): 116, 117
Drug grants: 55
Drug habit: 151
Drug law violation arrests
regional distribution (1981–93): 106, 107
Drug law violations: 103

Drug mentions: 166
Drug offenses
average length of drug felony sentences: 116, 117
federal drug convictions: 120
felony convictions in state courts (1992): 118
growing docket of cases: 119
handling of drug cases (1992): 108
number and percentage of inmates in state prisons
(1979–92): 112, 113
trends in categories of (1982–92): 111
trends in state prison admissions (1982–92): 110
Drug possession
average length of drug felony sentences: 116, 117
demographic characteristics: 114
federal drug convictions (1985–92): 120, 121
felony convictions in state courts (1992): 118
Drug sale/possession
drug use during (1990): 104
Drug smuggling
by mode of transportation (1986): 66, 67
Drug testing in the workplace
costs of drug use: 164
Drug testing programs in private business (1989): 94
Drug trafficking: 107
arrest statistics (1981–93): 106, 107
average length of drug felony sentences: 116, 117
demographic characteristics: 114, 115
drug use during (1990): 105
federal drug convictions (1985–92): 121
felony convictions in state courts (1992): 118, 119
multiagency task forces: 131
Drug treatment costs (1989): 177
donations: 176
federal government: 176
fees: 176
funding source: 176
local government: 176
private funding: 176
state government: 176
welfare: 176
Drug treatment program
as a demand reduction tactic: 125
Drug use
adolescents (1992): 17
among high school seniors (1991–94): 76
as a symptom: 79
casual: 73, 74, 75
cocaine use and overall illegal drug use trends (1979–
93): 70, 71
cocaine use trends (1972–92): 74, 75
DUI offenses: 38, 39
during crimes (1990): 104, 105

effects of: 78, 79

emergency room episodes (1988–93): 166, 167

estimated number of cocaine and heroin users (1988–93): 72

fatally injured drivers (1993): 22, 23

heavy: 73, 74, 75

illegal, individuals reporting (1993): 68, 69

murders in U.S. (1986–93): 98

safety hazards in workplace: 95

young adults during past month (1974–91): 88, 89

Drug Use Forecasting (DUF) program: 83, 105

Drug use sampling of past month (1992): 84

Drug-abuse treatment

census of clients in (1980–92): 172, 173

Drug-abuse treatment (1989–96): 174, 175

Drug-free school zones: 55

Drug-induced deaths

causes: 169

Drug-related arrests (1988–93): 102

Drug-related personal income amounts, monthly: 150

Drugs, schedules for: 54

Drunkenness: 40, 41

arrests for (1993): 42, 43

arrests in the U.S. (1993): 44, 45

DUF see Drug Use Forecasting Program

DUI see Driving Under the Influence

E

Ecuador

cocaine production (1992, 1993): 58

Education

cigarette smokers (1992): 184

women cigarette smokers: 187

Education levels

cigarette smokers (1992): 185

Embezzlement

drug use during (1990): 105

Emergency room episodes

drug use (1988–93): 166, 167

drug-related visits (1993): 170, 171

Emphysema

relative risks attributable to smoking (1990): 204

Employee assistance programs

costs of drug use: 164

Employment

alcohol use demographics (1991): 8, 9

Environmental smoke: 201

Equanil®

DEA ranking schedule: 80

Esophageal tumors

relative risks attributable to smoking (1990): 204, 205

Ethnic groups

alcohol use demographics (1991): 8, 9

cigarette smokers (1992): 184

Experimenters (smokers)

definition of: 191

F

FAS see Fetal alcohol syndrome

Fatalities in alcohol-related traffic accidents (1982–91): 24, 25

Fatally injured drunk drivers (1980–93): 30, 31

FBI see Federal Bureau of Investigation

Federal asset forfeiture funds (1986–90): 148

Federal Aviation Administration: 135

Federal Bureau of Investigation: 41, 103, 149

Federal Drug Control Legislation (1868–1990): 54, 55

Federal prisons, construction of: 149

Federal seizures of marijuana, cocaine, and heroin (1989–93): 132, 133

Felonies: 109

Felony convictions

in state courts (1992): 118, 119

Fetal alcohol syndrome (FAS)

rates (1979–93): 48, 49

Finance

drug testing programs (1989): 94

Financial instruments

seizure by the DEA (1992): 146

Fish and Wildlife Service: 141

Florida

cannabis eradication efforts (1990): 142

cigarette smokers aged 35 and over (1990): 182

deaths attributed to smoking (1990): 202

motor vehicle crash fatalities (1993): 20

potential years of life lost by cigarette smoking (1990): 200

Forgery

drug use during (1990): 104, 105

Former smokers

definition of: 191

Fort Lauderdale, FL

drug use by arrested persons (1991): 82

Fraud

drug use during (1990): 104, 105

felony convictions in state courts (1992): 118

G

Gangs
    drug use (1993–94) and: 86
Gender
    adolescent drinking and smoking (1992): 16, 17
    alcohol use by adolescents (1992): 14, 15
    alcohol use demographics (1991): 8, 9
    blood alcohol concentrations (BACs) of fatally injured
        drivers (1993): 22, 23
    cigarette smokers aged 35 and over by state (1990):
        182, 183
    cigarette smoking by youths aged 12–21 (1992): 190,
        191
    cocaine use by adolescents (1992): 14
    convicted drug felons: 114, 115
    deaths attributed to smoking (1990): 202, 203
    deaths induced by alcohol (1979–92): 50, 51
    drug use by adolescents (1992): 15
    drug use by arrested persons by city (1991): 82, 83
    drug use sampling of past month (1992): 84, 85
    drug-induced deaths (1979–92): 168, 169
    DUI arrests (1993): 36
    marijuana use by adolescents (1992): 14
    percentage of smokers aged 12–21: 190
    potential years of life lost by cigarette smoking (1990):
        200, 201
    relative risks attributable to smoking (1990): 204
    smokeless tobacco use: 193
    smokeless tobacco use by adolescents (1992): 14
    total arrests for DUI (1993): 38, 39
    women smokers aged 18–44 (1987–92): 186, 187
General Estimates System (GES) for the National
    Highway Traffic Safety Administration (NHTSA):
    27
Georgia
    cannabis eradication efforts (1990): 142
    cigarette smokers aged 35 and over (1990): 182
    deaths attributed to smoking (1990): 202
    motor vehicle crash fatalities (1993): 20
    potential years of life lost by cigarette smoking (1990):
        200
GES see General Estimates System for the National
    Highway Traffic Safety Administration
Guatemala
    opium production (1988–93): 60
Guns
    carried to school (1993–94), and drug use: 86

H

Hallucinogens
    individuals reporting drug use (1993): 68, 69
    use among high school seniors (1991–94): 76, 77
    use during past month (1974–91): 88
Hard-core users
    cocaine consumption (1972–92): 75
Harrison Narcotics Act: 54
Hashish
    DEA ranking schedule: 80
    international drug seizures (1989–93): 138, 139
    multiagency enforcement approach: 131
    THC content of seized (1975–90): 100
    use among high school seniors (1991–94): 76
    use during past month (1974–91): 88, 89
    worldwide production (1988–93): 64
Hawaii: 7
    cannabis eradication efforts (1990): 142, 143
    cannabis plant destruction (1982–90): 141
    cigarette smokers aged 35 and over (1990): 182
    deaths attributed to smoking (1990): 202
    drug abuse surveys: 7
    motor vehicle crash fatalities (1993): 20
    potential years of life lost by cigarette smoking (1990):
        200
Health care costs
    illegal drug use: 164
Health Care Financing Administration: 199
Heroin
    DEA ranking schedule: 80
    effects of: 78
    emergency room episodes (1988–93): 166, 167
    estimated number of users (1988–93): 72, 73
    federal seizures of (1989–93): 132, 133
    individuals reporting drug use (1993): 68, 69
    mind-altering effects of: 79
    multiagency enforcement approach: 131
    retail price per gram (1988–93): 156, 157
    smuggling, by mode of transportation (1986): 66, 67
    state and local narcotics enforcement (1990): 144
    trends of use (1972–92): 75
    U.S. expenditures on (1988–93): 152, 153
    use among high school seniors (1991–94): 76
    use by U.S. military personnel (1992): 92
    use during past month (1974–91): 88
Heroin Signature Report Program: 61
HIV see Human immuno deficiency virus
Hmong: 57
Home-health care
    cost of smoking-related sickness (1987): 198

Homeless
  drug abuse surveys: 7
Homicide
  alcohol involvement (1992): 46, 47
  costs to society from drug use: 164
  deaths in the workplace (1992): 97
  drug-related in U.S. (1986–93): 98, 99
  drug use during crimes (1990): 104
  in the workplace (1992): 96
Hospital care
  cost of smoking-related sickness (1987): 198, 199
Housing and Urban Development: 175
Houston, TX
  drug use by arrested persons (1991): 82
Human immuno deficiency virus (HIV)
  infection spread by injection: 157
Hypertensive diseases
  relative risks attributable to smoking (1990): 204

I

Idaho
  cannabis eradication efforts (1990): 142
  cigarette smokers aged 35 and over (1990): 182
  deaths attributed to smoking (1990): 202
  motor vehicle crash fatalities (1993): 20
  potential years of life lost by cigarette smoking (1990): 200
Illegal drug crops
  world production of (1987–91): 56
Illegal drug use
  cocaine use trends (1979–93): 70, 71
  costs to society: 164, 165, 177
  individuals reporting (1993): 68, 69
Illegal drugs
  effects of: 79
  total U.S. expenditures (1988–93): 152, 153
  use during past month (1974–91): 88
Illinois
  cannabis eradication efforts (1990): 142
  cigarette smokers aged 35 and over (1990): 182
  deaths attributed to smoking (1990): 202
  motor vehicle crash fatalities (1993): 20
  potential years of life lost by cigarette smoking (1990): 200
Immigration and Naturalization Service: 149
Immigration and Naturalization Service's Border Patrol: 135
Importation
  federal drug convictions (1985–92): 120, 121
Imprisonment
  as a demand reduction tactic: 125
  average length of drug felony sentences: 116, 117
India
  marijuana production (1988–93): 63
Indiana
  cannabis plant destruction (1982–90): 141
  cigarette smokers aged 35 and over (1990): 182
  deaths attributed to smoking (1990): 202
  motor vehicle crash fatalities (1993): 20
  potential years of life lost by cigarette smoking (1990): 200
Indianapolis, IN
  drug use by arrested persons (1991): 82
Infant disease
  relative risks attributable to smoking (1990): 205
Infant mortality
  cigarette smokers and: 187
Influenza
  relative risks attributable to smoking (1990): 204
Inhalants: 89
  use among high school seniors (1991–94): 76, 77
  use by U.S. military personnel (1992): 92
  use during past month (1974–91): 88
Insurance
  drug testing programs (1989): 94
Interdiction
  definition: 135
Internal Revenue Service: 149
International drug seizures
  decline in: 139
International drug seizures (1989–93): 138, 139
International Opium Convention: 54
Iowa
  cannabis eradication efforts (1990): 142
  cigarette smokers aged 35 and over (1990): 182
  deaths attributed to smoking (1990): 202
  motor vehicle crash fatalities (1993): 20
  potential years of life lost by cigarette smoking (1990): 200
Iran: 61
  world opium supply: 57, 61
IRS see Internal Revenue Service
Ischemic heart disease: 204

J

Jamaica
  marijuana production (1988–93): 62
  marijuana supplier: 57
  wholesale prices for marijuana (1991): 160, 161
Justice Department: 175

K

Kansas
    cannabis eradication efforts (1990): 142
    cigarette smokers aged 35 and over (1990): 182
    deaths attributed to smoking (1990): 202
    motor vehicle crash fatalities (1993): 20
    potential years of life lost by cigarette smoking (1990): 200

Kansas City, MO
    drug use by arrested persons (1991): 82

Kentucky
    cannabis eradication efforts (1990): 142
    cigarette smokers aged 35 and over (1990): 182, 183
    deaths attributed to smoking (1990): 202
    motor vehicle crash fatalities (1993): 20
    potential years of life lost by cigarette smoking (1990): 200

Kidney, tumors of
    relative risks attributable to smoking (1990): 204

Kurds: 57

L

Laboratories
    seizures of illegal drug (1975–91): 136, 137

Laboratory seizures
    as supply reduction tactics: 125

Land and marine seizures of marijuana and cocaine (1976–92): 134, 135

Land border interdiction: 135

Laos
    marijuana production (1988–93): 63
    opium production (1988–93): 60
    world opium supply: 57

Larceny
    drug use during crimes (1990): 104
    felony convictions in state courts (1992): 118

Larceny-theft
    drug use during (1990): 105

Larynx tumors
    relative risks attributable to smoking (1990): 204

Lebanon
    hashish production (1988–93): 64, 65
    opium production (1988–93): 60

Legal income: 151

Legal intoxication level: 47

Librium®
    DEA ranking schedule: 80

Licensed drivers, number of: 41

Lip tumors
    relative risks attributable to smoking (1990): 204, 205

Liquor
    role in violent behavior in youth (1993–94): 86

Liquor law violations: 40, 41

Lomotil®
    DEA ranking schedule: 80

Los Angeles, CA
    cocaine, retail price per gram (1986–91): 158
    drug use by arrested persons (1991): 82

Lost productivity costs
    illegal drug use: 164

Louisiana
    cannabis eradication efforts (1990): 142
    cigarette smokers aged 35 and over (1990): 182
    deaths attributed to smoking (1990): 202
    motor vehicle crash fatalities (1993): 20
    potential years of life lost by cigarette smoking (1990): 200
    results of surveys on effective strategies to prevent teenage smoking (1993): 208, 209
    surveys on prohibition or restriction of cigarette smoking (1993): 206

LSD see Lysergic acid diethylamide

Lung cancer
    women cigarette smokers and: 187

Lung tumors
    relative risks attributable to smoking (1990): 204

Lysergic acid diethylamide (LSD)
    DEA ranking schedule: 80
    drug laboratory seizures (1975–91): 137
    effects of: 78
    state and local narcotics enforcement (1990): 144
    use among high school seniors (1991–94): 76
    use by U.S. military personnel (1992): 92

M

Maine
    cannabis eradication efforts (1990): 142
    cigarette smokers aged 35 and over (1990): 182
    deaths attributed to smoking (1990): 202
    motor vehicle crash fatalities (1993): 20
    potential years of life lost by cigarette smoking (1990): 200

Manhattan, NY
    drug use by arrested persons (1991): 82, 83

Manufacture
    federal drug convictions (1985–92): 120, 121

Marijuana: 82, 83, 84, 85, 89
    adolescent use: 191

DEA ranking schedule: 80
deaths in the workplace (1992): 96
effects of: 78
emergency room episodes (1988–93): 166, 167
federal seizures of (1989–93): 132, 133
individuals reporting drug use (1993): 68, 69
land and marine seizures (1976–92): 134, 135
mind-altering effects of: 79
multiagency enforcement approach: 131
processing and refining: 57
role in violent behavior in youth (1993–94): 86
smuggling, by mode of transportation (1986): 66, 67
state and local narcotics enforcement (1990): 144, 145
THC content of seized (1975–90): 100
U.S. expenditures on (1988–93): 152, 153
use among high school seniors (1991–94): 76, 77
use by adolescents (1992): 14
use by U.S. military personnel (1992): 92
use during crimes (1990): 104, 105
use during past month (1974–91): 88
wholesale prices for (1991): 160, 161
world production of (1987–91): 56
worldwide production (1988–93): 62, 63
Marijuana Tax Act: 54
Marijuana/hashish
international drug seizures (1989–93): 138, 139
Marine Corps: 93
drug use (1992): 92, 93
Marine interdiction: 135
Maryland
cannabis eradication efforts (1990): 143
cigarette smokers aged 35 and over (1990): 182
deaths attributed to smoking (1990): 202
motor vehicle crash fatalities (1993): 20
potential years of life lost by cigarette smoking (1990): 200
Massachusetts
cannabis eradication efforts (1990): 142
cigarette smokers aged 35 and over (1990): 182
deaths attributed to smoking (1990): 202
motor vehicle crash fatalities (1993): 20
potential years of life lost by cigarette smoking (1990): 200
Medicaid
cost of smoking-related sickness (1987): 198, 199
Medical care
costs of smoking-related sickness (1987): 198, 199
Medicare
cost of smoking-related sickness (1987): 198, 199
Mental Health Centers Act amendments: 54
Methadone: 82
DEA ranking schedule: 80

deaths in the workplace (1992): 96
use during crimes (1990): 104, 105
Methamphetamine
drug laboratory seizures (1975–91): 136
multiagency enforcement approach: 131
Methaqualone: 82
DEA ranking schedule: 80
drug laboratory seizures (1975–91): 137
multiagency enforcement approach: 131
U.S. expenditures on (1988–93): 153
use among high school seniors (1991–94): 76, 77
use during crimes (1990): 104, 105
Mexico
drug smuggling to U.S.: 67
marijuana production (1988–93): 62, 63
marijuana supplier: 57
opium production (1988–93): 60
wholesale prices for marijuana (1991): 160, 161
world opium supply: 61
Miami, FL
cocaine retail price per gram (1986–91): 158
drug use by arrested persons (1991): 82, 83
Michigan
cannabis eradication efforts (1990): 142
cigarette smokers aged 35 and over (1990): 182
deaths attributed to smoking (1990): 202
motor vehicle crash fatalities (1993): 20
potential years of life lost by cigarette smoking (1990): 200
Middle East
drug smuggling to U.S.: 67
Military personnel
drug abuse surveys: 7
Miltown®
DEA ranking schedule: 80
Minimum age 21 drinking laws: 35
Mining
drug testing programs (1989): 94
Minnesota
cannabis eradication efforts (1990): 142
cigarette smokers aged 35 and over (1990): 182
deaths attributed to smoking (1990): 202
motor vehicle crash fatalities (1993): 20
potential years of life lost by smoking (1990): 200
Misdemeanors: 109
Mississippi
cannabis eradication efforts (1990): 142
cigarette smokers aged 35 and over (1990): 182
deaths attributed to smoking (1990): 202
motor vehicle crash fatalities (1993): 20
potential years of life lost by cigarette smoking (1990): 200

Missouri
    cannabis eradication efforts (1990): 142
    cannabis plant destruction (1982–90): 141
    cigarette smokers aged 35 and over (1990): 182
    deaths attributed to smoking (1990): 202
    motor vehicle crash fatalities (1993): 20
    potential years of life lost by cigarette smoking (1990): 200
    results of surveys on effective strategies to prevent teenage smoking (1993): 208, 209
    surveys on prohibition or restriction of cigarette smoking (1993): 206
Money laundering cases: 149
Money laundering laws: 147
Montana
    cannabis eradication efforts (1990): 142, 143
    cigarette smokers aged 35 and over (1990): 182
    deaths attributed to smoking (1990): 202
    motor vehicle crash fatalities (1993): 20
    potential years of life lost by cigarette smoking (1990): 200
    smokeless tobacco use: 193
Morocco
    hashish production (1988–93): 64, 65
Morphine: 61
    DEA ranking schedule: 80
    deaths in the workplace (1992): 96
Mortality
    alcohol-induced deaths (1979–92): 50, 51
    cigarette smoking and: 202, 203
    drug use in the workplace (1992): 96
    drug-induced deaths by gender (1979–92): 168, 169
    drug-related accidents in the workplace: 164
    drug-related murders in U.S. (1986–93): 98, 99
    fatal workplace injuries involving alcohol (1992): 46, 47
    fatally injured drunk drivers (1980–93): 30, 31
    youth crash fatalities (1982–93): 32, 33
    youth crash fatality rate (1982–93): 34
    youth crash fatality rate and alcohol (1982–93): 35
Motor vehicle theft
    drug use during (1990): 105
Multiagency drug enforcement task forces (1990): 130, 131
Murder
    drug-related in U.S. (1986–93): 98, 99
    felony convictions in state courts (1992): 118, 119

N

Narcotic Addict Treatment Act: 54

Narcotic Drugs Import and Export Act: 54
Narcotic Drugs Laws: 98
Narcotics Addict Rehabilitation Act: 54
Narcotics Control Act: 54
National Cancer Institute: 209
National Cancer Institute's Community Intervention Trial for Smoking Cessation: 207
National Center for Health Statistics: 17
National Drug Enforcement Policy Board: 55
National Drug Treatment Unit Survey (NDATUS): 177
National Guard: 141
National Health Interview Survey of Youth Risk Behavior: 15
National Health Interview Survey—Cancer Control and Epidemiology Supplements (NHIS-CCES): 185
National Health Objectives for the Year 2000: 191
National Highway Traffic Safety Administration (NHTSA): 25, 33, 35, 47
National Household Survey on Drug Abuse (NHSDA) (1993): 69
National Institute of Justice: 83
National Institute on Drug Abuse: 5, 7, 9, 13, 54, 175, 189
National Park Service: 141
National Survey on Drug Abuse: 7
Navy
    drug use (1992): 92, 93
NDATUS see National Drug Treatment Unit Survey
Nebraska
    cannabis eradication efforts (1990): 142
    cannabis plant destruction (1982–90): 141
    cigarette smokers aged 35 and over (1990): 182
    deaths attributed to smoking (1990): 202
    motor vehicle crash fatalities (1993): 20
    potential years of life lost by cigarette smoking (1990): 200
Negotiable instruments
    seizure by DEA (1992): 147
Neoplasms
    relative risks attributable to smoking (1990): 205
Neoplasms (tumors): 204
Nepal
    marijuana production (1988–93): 63
Nevada
    cannabis eradication efforts (1990): 143
    cigarette smokers aged 35 and over (1990): 182
    deaths attributed to smoking (1990): 202, 203
    motor vehicle crash fatalities (1993): 20

potential years of life lost by cigarette smoking (1990): 200

Never smokers
definition of: 191

New Hampshire
cannabis eradication efforts (1990): 143
cigarette smokers aged 35 and over (1990): 182
deaths attributed to smoking (1990): 202
motor vehicle crash fatalities (1993): 20
potential years of life lost by cigarette smoking (1990): 200

New Jersey
cannabis eradication efforts (1990): 143
cigarette smokers aged 35 and over (1990): 182
deaths attributed to smoking (1990): 202
motor vehicle crash fatalities (1993): 20
potential years of life lost by cigarette smoking (1990): 200
results of surveys on effective strategies to prevent teenage smoking (1993): 208
surveys on prohibition or restriction of cigarette smoking (1993): 206

New Mexico
cannabis eradication efforts (1990): 142
cigarette smokers aged 35 and over (1990): 182
deaths attributed to smoking (1990): 202
motor vehicle crash fatalities (1993): 20
potential years of life lost by cigarette smoking (1990): 200

New Orleans, LA
drug use by arrested persons (1991): 82

New York
cannabis eradication efforts (1990): 142
cigarette smokers aged 35 and over (1990): 182
cocaine, retail price per gram (1986–91): 158
deaths attributed to smoking (1990): 202
motor vehicle crash fatalities (1993): 20
potential years of life lost by cigarette smoking (1990): 200

NHIS-CCES see National Health Interview Survey—Cancer Control and Epidemiology Supplements

NHSDA see National Household Survey on Drug Abuse

NHTSA see National Highway Traffic Safety Administration

Nicotine
reasons for use (1993): 195

Nicotine addiction: 195, 197

Nicotine withdrawal symptoms
reported by teenagers (1993): 196, 197

North America
opium production (1988–93): 60

North Carolina
cannabis eradication efforts (1990): 142
cigarette smokers aged 35 and over (1990): 182
deaths attributed to smoking (1990): 202
motor vehicle crash fatalities (1993): 21
potential years of life lost by cigarette smoking (1990): 200

North Dakota
cannabis eradication efforts (1990): 143
cigarette smokers aged 35 and over (1990): 182, 183
deaths attributed to smoking (1990): 202
motor vehicle crash fatalities (1993): 21
potential years of life lost by cigarette smoking (1990): 200

Nursing-home care
cost of smoking-related sickness (1987): 198, 199

O

OCDETF see Organized Crime Drug Enforcement Task Force

Offenses
average length of drug felony sentences: 116, 117
felony convictions in state courts (1992): 118, 119
trends in categories of (1982–92): 110
trends in the categories of: 113

Office for Substance Abuse Prevention (OSAP): 55

Office of National Drug Abuse Policy: 55

Office of National Drug Control Policy: 59, 75, 125, 149

Office on Smoking and Health: 205

Ohio
cannabis eradication efforts (1990): 142
cigarette smokers aged 35 and over (1990): 182, 183
deaths attributed to smoking (1990): 202
motor vehicle crash fatalities (1993): 21
potential years of life lost by cigarette smoking (1990): 200
results of surveys on effective strategies to prevent teenage smoking (1993): 208
surveys on prohibition or restriction of cigarette smoking (1993): 206

Oklahoma
cannabis eradication efforts (1990): 142
cigarette smokers aged 35 and over (1990): 182, 183
deaths attributed to smoking (1990): 202
motor vehicle crash fatalities (1993): 21
potential years of life lost by cigarette smoking (1990): 200
results of surveys on effective strategies to prevent teenage smoking (1993): 208, 209

surveys on prohibition or restriction of cigarette
smoking (1993): 206
Omaha, NE
drug use by arrested persons (1991): 82, 83
Opiates: 82
international drug seizures (1989–93): 138, 139
use among high school seniors (1991–94): 76, 77
use during crimes (1990): 104
Opium: 54
processing and refining: 57
world production of (1987–91): 56
worldwide production (1988–93): 60, 61
Opium Exclusion Act: 54
Opium Poppy Control Act: 54
Oral cavity tumors
relative risks attributable to smoking (1990): 204, 205
Oregon
cannabis eradication efforts (1990): 142
cigarette smokers aged 35 and over (1990): 183
deaths attributed to smoking (1990): 202
motor vehicle crash fatalities (1993): 21
potential years of life lost by cigarette smoking (1990):
200
Organized Crime Drug Enforcement Task Force
(OCDETF): 131
OSAP see Office for Substance Abuse Prevention
Overdose
emergency room episodes (1993): 170

P

P2P
drug laboratory seizures (1975–91): 137
Pakistan
hashish production (1988–93): 64, 65
marijuana production (1988–93): 63
opium production (1988–93): 60
world opium supply: 57
Panama
marijuana production (1988–93): 63
Pancreatic tumors
relative risks attributable to smoking (1990): 204
PCP see Phencyclidine
Pennsylvania
cannabis eradication efforts (1990): 142
cigarette smokers aged 35 and over (1990): 183
deaths attributed to smoking (1990): 203
motor vehicle crash fatalities (1993): 21
potential years of life lost by cigarette smoking (1990):
201
Peru: 57

coca leaf and opium supplier: 57
cocaine production: 59
cocaine production (1992, 1993): 58
wholesale cocaine prices (1991): 162, 163
Pharmaceutical industry, regulation of the: 54
Pharmacy Act: 54
Pharynx neoplasms
relative risks attributable to smoking (1990): 204, 205
Phencyclidine (PCP): 82, 89
DEA ranking schedule: 80
drug laboratory seizures (1975–91): 136, 137
multiagency enforcement approach: 131
state and local narcotics enforcement (1990): 144
use among high school seniors (1991–94): 76, 77
use by U.S. military personnel (1992): 92
use during crimes (1990): 104, 105
use during past month (1974–91): 88
Phenobarbital
DEA ranking schedule: 80
Philadelphia, PA
drug use by arrested persons (1991): 82
Phoenix, AZ
drug use by arrested persons (1991): 82
Physician care
cost of smoking-related sickness (1987): 198, 199
Pneumonia
relative risks attributable to smoking (1990): 204
Police
youth trouble and drug use (1993–94): 86, 87
Police protection
enforcement of narcotics laws (1990): 128, 129
multiagency drug enforcement task forces: 130, 131
state and local spending: 127
state and local spending (1991): 126
Poppy/opium
international drug seizures (1989–93): 138, 139
Porter Narcotic Farm Act: 54
Portland, OR
drug use by arrested persons (1991): 82
Precursor chemicals, regulation of: 55
Pregnancy
cigarette smoking risk: 187
fetal alcohol syndrome rates (1979–93): 48, 49
Premature death
cigarette smoking and: 201
cigarette smoking as cause of: 203
Prescription drugs
cost of smoking-related sickness (1987): 198
PRIDE USA Survey, 1993–94: 87
Private insurance
cost of smoking-related sickness (1987): 198

Property offenses
 felony convictions in state courts (1992): 118
 handling of drug cases (1992): 108
 trends in state prison admissions: 113
 trends in state prison admissions (1982–92): 110
Propoxyphene: 82
 use during crimes (1990): 104, 105
Prostitution
 drug use during (1990): 104, 105
Psychotherapeutic drugs
 mind-altering effects of: 79
 use during past month (1974–91): 88
Public assistance: 151
Public order offenses
 trends in state prison admissions: 110, 113
Puerto Rico
 legal drinking age: 7
 marijuana supplier: 57
Pure Food and Drug Act: 54

R

Race
 alcohol use demographics (1991): 8, 9
 cigarette smokers (1992): 184
 convicted drug felons: 114, 115
Ranking specific drugs: 81
Rape
 felony convictions in state courts (1992): 118
Real property
 seizure by the DEA (1992): 146
Research Triangle Institute: 93
Respiratory diseases
 relative risks attributable to smoking (1990): 204, 205
 women cigarette smokers and: 187
Respiratory distress syndrome
 relative risks attributable to smoking (1990): 205
Retail trade
 drug testing programs (1989): 94
Rhode Island
 cannabis eradication efforts (1990): 143
 cigarette smokers aged 35 and over (1990): 183
 deaths attributed to smoking (1990): 203
 motor vehicle crash fatalities (1993): 21
 potential years of life lost by cigarette smoking (1990): 201
Robbery
 costs to society from drug use: 164
 drug use during (1990): 104, 105
 felony convictions in state courts (1992): 118
Robitussin AC®

DEA ranking schedule: 80
Rural drug enforcement: 55
Russia
 marijuana production (1988–93): 63

S

San Antonio, TX
 drug use by arrested persons (1991): 82, 83
San Diego, CA
 drug use by arrested persons (1991): 82, 83
San Jose, CA
 drug use by arrested persons (1991): 82
Schedule I drug: 81
Schedule V drug: 81
Scheduling of drugs: 80, 81
Second-hand smoke: 207
Securities
 seizure by DEA (1992): 147
Sedatives
 mind-altering effects of: 79
 use among high school seniors (1991–94): 76
Sinsemilla
 destruction of plants (1982–90): 141
 seizure of: 143
 THC content (1975–90): 100, 101
Smokeless tobacco
 adolescent use: 191
 use by teenagers (1986–94): 192, 193
Snuff *see* Tobacco (smokeless)
Socioeconomic status
 cigarette smokers (1992): 184, 185
 women smokers aged 18–44 (1987–92): 186
South America
 drug smuggling to U.S.: 67
 opium production (1988–93): 60
 world opium supply: 61
South Carolina
 cannabis eradication efforts (1990): 142
 cigarette smokers aged 35 and over (1990): 183
 deaths attributed to smoking (1990): 203
 motor vehicle crash fatalities (1993): 21
 potential years of life lost by cigarette smoking (1990): 201
 results of surveys on effective strategies to prevent teenage smoking (1993): 208
 surveys on prohibition or restriction of cigarette smoking (1993): 206
South Dakota
 cannabis eradication efforts (1990): 142
 cigarette smokers aged 35 and over (1990): 183

deaths attributed to smoking (1990): 203
motor vehicle crash fatalities (1993): 21
potential years of life lost by cigarette smoking (1990):
    201
Southeast Asia
    opium production (1988–93): 60
    world opium supply: 57, 61
Southwest Asia
    opium production (1988–93): 60
    world opium supply: 61
St. Louis, MO
    drug use by arrested persons (1991): 82
State and local narcotics enforcement (1990): 144,
    145
Statistical leakage or bleeding: 37
Steroid use
    desired effects: 91
    high school seniors (1989–94): 90, 91
Stimulants: 54
    mind-altering effects of: 79
    state and local narcotics enforcement (1990): 144
    use among high school seniors (1991–94): 76, 77
Stolen property
    drug use during crimes (1990): 104, 105
Stolen vehicle
    drug use during crimes (1990): 104
Substance Abuse and Mental Health Services
    Administration: 3, 175
Sudden infant death syndrome
    relative risks attributable to smoking (1990): 205
Suicide: 47
    alcohol involvement (1992): 46, 47
    deaths in the workplace (1992): 97
    drug use (1993–94) and thoughts of: 86, 87
    in the workplace (1992): 96
Supply reduction tactics: 125
Surgeon General's Report: 15, 17

T

Talwin®
    DEA ranking schedule: 80
TAPS-II see Teenage Attitudes and Practices Survey
Taxation: 55
Teenage Attitudes and Practices Survey (TAPS-II),
    1993: 194, 196
Tennessee
    cannabis eradication efforts (1990): 142
    cannabis plant destruction (1982–90): 141
    cigarette smokers aged 35 and over (1990): 183

deaths attributed to smoking (1990): 203
motor vehicle crash fatalities (1993): 21
potential years of life lost by cigarette smoking (1990):
    201
Tetrahydrocannabinol (THC) content: 65
    of seized marijuana (1975–90): 100
Tetrahydrocannabinol content of seized marijuana
    (1975–90): 100, 101
Texas
    cannabis eradication efforts (1990): 142
    cigarette smokers aged 35 and over (1990): 183
    deaths attributed to smoking (1990): 203
    motor vehicle crash fatalities (1993): 21
    potential years of life lost by cigarette smoking (1990):
        201
    results of surveys on effective strategies to prevent
        teenage smoking (1993): 208
    surveys on prohibition or restriction of cigarette
        smoking (1993): 206
Thailand
    marijuana production (1988–93): 63
    opium production (1988–93): 60
    wholesale prices for marijuana (1991): 160, 161
    world opium supply: 57
THC see tetrahydrocannabinol content
Theft
    costs to society from drug use: 164
    drug use during (1990): 104
Threatening harm
    drug use (1993–94) and: 86, 87
Tobacco
    adolescents' use of (1992): 16, 17
    cigarette smokers aged 35 and over by state (1990):
        182, 183
    cigarette smoking by high school seniors (1975–94):
        188, 189
    cigarette smoking by youths aged 12–21 (1992): 190,
        191
    cigarette consumption per capita (1900–94): 180, 181
    deaths attributed to smoking (1990): 202, 203
    medical care costs for smoking-related sickness
        (1987): 198, 199
    nicotine withdrawal symptoms reported by teenagers
        (1993): 196, 197
    reasons for using cigarettes (1993): 194, 195
    relative risks attributable to smoking (1990): 204
    survey results on effective strategies to prevent
        teenage smoking (1993): 208, 209
    survey results on prohibiting or restricting smoking
        (1993): 206, 207
    use of as transition: 69
    use within the U.S.: 185

women smokers aged 18–44 (1987–92): 186, 187

years of life lost due to smoking (1990): 200, 201

Tobacco (smokeless)

adolescents (1992): 17

use by adolescents (1992): 14

use by teenagers (1986–94): 192, 193

Total drug episodes: 167

Total drug mentions: 167

Toxicology reports: 97

Tracheal tumors

relative risks attributable to smoking (1990): 204

Trafficking, penalties for: 55

Tranquilizers: 92

mind-altering effects of: 79

use among high school seniors (1991–94): 76, 77

use by U.S. military personnel: 93

Transportation

drug testing programs (1989): 94

Turkey: 61

government control of opium supply: 61

U

U.S.

drug smuggling (1986): 66, 67

hashish production (1988–93): 65

marijuana production (1988–93): 63

drug use by arrested persons (1991): 82

U.S. Coast Guard

preventing marine drug smuggling: 135

U.S. Criminal Justice System

expenditures on drug-related crime: 164

federal drug control spending (1995–96): 124, 125

handling of drug cases (1992): 108, 109

handling of drug cases: 119

supply-side targeting: 121

U.S. Customs Service

interdicting land border smuggling: 135

marijuana and cocaine seizures (1976–92): 134

U.S. Department of Defense

Authorization Act: 54

drug use (1992): 92, 93, 135, 141, 175

U.S. Department of Health and Human Services: 3, 177, 191

U.S. Department of Justice: 149

Asset Forfeiture Fund: 125, 149

U.S. Department of Transportation: 23, 25

drug testing of employees: 95

U.S. Department of Veterans Affairs: 175

U.S. Forest Service: 141

U.S. Marshals Service: 149

U.S. National Health Interview Survey, 1987–92: 186

U.S. Postal Inspection Service: 149

U.S. Surgeon General: 181

University of California: 199

University of Michigan's Institute for Social Research: 13

Urinary bladder, tumors of

relative risks attributable to smoking (1990): 204

Utah

cannabis eradication efforts (1990): 143

cigarette smokers aged 35 and over (1990): 183

deaths attributed to smoking (1990): 203

motor vehicle crash fatalities (1993): 21

potential years of life lost by cigarette smoking (1990): 201

V

Vagrancy: 40, 41

Vehicles

seizure by the DEA (1992): 146

Vermont

cannabis eradication efforts (1990): 142

cigarette smokers aged 35 and over (1990): 183

deaths attributed to smoking (1990): 203

motor vehicle crash fatalities (1993): 21

potential years of life lost by cigarette smoking (1990): 201

Vessels

seizure by the DEA (1992): 146

Vietnam

marijuana production (1988–93): 63

Violent behavior

liquor and marijuana use and role among youth (1993–94): 86, 87

Violent Crime Control and Law Enforcement Act of 1994: 175

Violent offenses

felony convictions in state courts (1992): 118, 119

handling of drug cases (1992): 108

trends in state prison admissions: 110

Virginia

cannabis eradication efforts (1990): 142

cigarette smokers aged 35 and over (1990): 183

deaths attributed to smoking (1990): 203

motor vehicle crash fatalities (1993): 21

potential years of life lost by cigarette smoking (1990): 201

Volsted Act: 54